Boarding Time

A Psychiatry Candidate's Guide to
Part II of the ABPN Examination

Second Edition

Boarding Time

A Psychiatry Candidate's Guide to Part II of the ABPN Examination

Second Edition

James Morrison, M.D.
Chief, Psychiatry Service
Department of Veterans Affairs
Northern California Health Care system
Martinez, California
Professor of Psychiatry
University of California, Davis

and

Rodrigo A. Muñoz, M.D.
Clinical Professor of Psychiatry
University of California, San Diego
Vice President
American Psychiatric Association

Washington, DC
London, England

Note. The authors have worked to ensure that all information in this book concerning drug dosages, schedules, and routes of administration is accurate as of the time of publication and consistent with standards set by the U.S. Food and Drug Administration and the general medical community. As medical research and practice advance, however, therapeutic standards may change. For this reason and because human and mechanical errors sometimes occur, we recommend that readers follow the advice of a physician who is directly involved in their care or the care of a member of their family.

Books published by the American Psychiatric Press, Inc., represent the views and opinions of the individual authors and do not necessarily represent the policies and opinions of the Press or the American Psychiatric Association.

Copyright © 1996 American Psychiatric Press, Inc.
ALL RIGHTS RESERVED
Manufactured in the United States of America on acid-free paper
99 98 97 96   4 3 2 1
First Edition

American Psychiatric Press, Inc.
1400 K Street, N.W., Washington, DC   20005

Library of Congress Cataloging-in-Publication Data
Morrison, James R., 1940-
    Boarding time: a psychiatry candidate's guide to part II of the
ABPN examination / James Morrison and Rodrigo A. Muñoz. — 2nd ed.
      p.   cm.
    ISBN 0-88048-722-4 (alk. paper)
    1. Psychiatrists—United States—Examinations—Study guides.
2. Psychiatry—Examinations—Study guides.   I. Muñoz, Rodrigo A.
II. Title.
    [DNLM: 1. Psychiatry—United States.   2. Specialty Boards—United
States.   3. Educational Measurement—methods.   WM 21 M879b 1996]
RC343.5.M67   1996
616.89′0076—dc20
DNLM/DLC
for Library of Congress   95-34139
                                                                        CIP

British Library Cataloguing in Publication Data
A CIP record is available from the British Library.

Contents

Preface to the Second Edition

Several factors have necessitated a second edition of *Boarding Time*. Here are some of them:

- Changes in fees and other details of the examination process
- New terminology with the adoption of DSM-IV
- New study materials available to candidates
- Helpful criticisms from readers of the first edition

Of course, much remains the same—the anxiety of the candidates, the reasons for failure, the fundamental approach to the patients, and—always—the benefits of practice. But in several areas we have updated and expanded *Boarding Time*.

In Chapters 4 and 5, we have updated our explanation of the examination process, reflecting (relatively) minor changes in the examinees' and examiners' information booklets. In Chapter 9 we have somewhat simplified and clarified the process of case formulation. In a completely new Chapter 13, we present in its entirety a mock board interview, including discussions the two examiners had about and with the candidate. Appendixes B and C have been substantially rewritten to conform to changes in Board eligibility. Appendix G is an all-new discussion of the specter of recertification. Throughout all text and tables, we have reflected the changes introduced by DSM-IV. Finally, we have updated Appendix E to give you a current list of suggested readings for further study.

Several examiners deserve our thanks for their contribution to the second edition. They include Drs. Irwin Feinberg, Rita Hargrave, and Mark Servis and a number of others who have requested anonymity. We also want to thank the candidate and the patient who so generously permitted us to record and use the mock board examination that appears as Chapter 13.

Preface to the First Edition

Why should you become certified? Why should any psychiatrist? Board certification is really just another phase in your psychiatric education, a process that may have begun a decade ago and that may continue another 40 years or more. You may be taking this step to earn more pay (as is true for some salaried positions) or to qualify for advancement in certain other jobs. Or perhaps your motivation is simply that Board certification is increasingly being regarded as a symbol of excellence.

But your certification is also important for our profession. When more psychiatrists have negotiated this hurdle in their training, all of us can present a stronger front to other physicians and to our patients. It will also allow us to press our case for better psychiatric insurance coverage to legislators and employers.

All medical specialties have Boards. Some rely exclusively on written exercises, sometimes augmented by videotape, to test the mettle of their candidates. A number of Boards use some form of oral exam. But in addition to the basic issues in psychiatry, which can be learned from textbooks, journals, and lectures, the practicing psychiatrist needs skills of quite a different nature.

We agree with the overwhelming majority of certified psychiatrists today, who believe that these skills can be adequately assessed only in the format of the live patient interview.

We also believe that Part II of the ABPN examination represents one of the most stressful events of the psychiatrist's professional life. During this ordeal the physician must put away the mantle of authority and wear the hair shirt of a witnessed interview. Within a rigid time limit the candidate must acquire a body of information and, still in the spotlight's glare, must formulate and defend a diagnosis, discuss such arcane subjects as etiology and prognosis, and finally, recommend and discuss therapy.

The ABPN serves the public, not candidates. Its function is evaluative, not educational, so it is not prepared to offer the assistance candidates require. This help must come from individuals and from organizations such as psychiatric training programs and the American Psychiatric Association (APA). The APA encourages its District branches to offer mock examinations; at annual meetings it sponsors discussions of a host of issues related to certification.

Boarding Time

This manual also aims to help physicians preparing for this examination to succeed. It is a manual of advice, not a scientific treatise. If there were more studies that bear on the problem of Board certification, we would have gladly reported them, but there are not. Therefore, much of what we have included is opinion — the opinion of examiners, of Board members, of candidates, and especially of the authors. But what we have written does not constitute the official opinion of either the American Board of Psychiatry and Neurology or of the APA.

We have tried at every juncture to separate fact from opinion in the text. We have tried to indicate by quotations that statements of examiners are their own opinions. They are generally opinions that we share, but we ask you to keep in mind that the opinions expressed here are not shared by all examiners and Board members. We present what others have told us worked for them. We believe that the suggestions will work for you.

Here's how we think this book can help you best:

If you are just beginning your preparation for the Boards, first read straight through *Boarding Time: A Psychiatry Candidate's Guide to Part II of the ABPN Examination*. Then, as you progress in your studies, go back to review any chapters you consider your weak areas.

If time is too short to read this entire book, or if you feel you are already well prepared and have taken one or more mock board exams, you might want to start with the chapters that deal with the mechanics of the Boards. They are Chapters 3, 4, 5, 6, and 11.

And if you have already unsuccessfully taken Part II and are trying to decide what to do next, start with Chapter 12. It suggests what specific steps you should and should not take.

Most books are created with the assistance of many people and this one is no exception. We are grateful to the numerous candidates, both successful and unsuccessful, who spent hours reliving their experiences with the Boards. We have retold many of their stories to emphasize important points. (All names and other identifying data have been altered to protect candidates' anonymity.)

Many examiners have also given generously of their time to help us identify and synthesize the characteristics that constitute a successful candidacy. In this respect we particularly want to thank Drs. Sid Zisook, Robert Moore, Hamp Atkinson, Charles Rabiner, and Igor Grant.

Of several (anonymous) reviewers for the American Psychiatric Press, two stand out as having spent hours commenting on drafts of our manuscript.

We also thank Mary Morrison, whose painstaking, thoughtful criticism helped clarify and condense many passages of text that might otherwise have remained obscure.

We greatly appreciate the time spent by the ABPN staff assisting us by collecting information from the public domain.

But while acknowledging the invaluable contributions of all these people, we hasten to claim for ourselves full responsibility for any remaining errors of fact or infelicities of expression.

Chapter 1 ——————————————————

Why Candidates Fail

To the uninitiated, it must seem easy. After all, Part II of the ABPN for psychiatrists involves nothing more than two hour-long sessions—one videotape and one live patient interview—each including a half-hour question-and-answer period conducted by two Board-certified psychiatrists. The problems presented are clinical ones; the questions posed are those the average clinician might expect to encounter in practice any day. Yet year after year, nearly half the candidates who take this oral examination fail it. Why is this so?

In gathering material for this book, we interviewed examiners and Board candidates alike to answer this question. We heard many answers and recorded many anecdotes. Although they seem numerous and varied at first, most boil down to a matter of inadequate preparation. This chapter documents and explains what that means, so that you can avoid some of the traps other candidates have fallen into.

Anatomy of a Board Casualty

When a candidate fails, it usually isn't because of a single error or deficiency. Most candidates who fail made a number of errors in gathering their facts or in interpreting the material presented by the patient or videotape. Here is how some of these problems piled up on one examinee.

> Several years out of residency, Dr. Wilson felt confident about the Part II examination. As a resident, Dr. Wilson had done well on the PRITE (Psychiatry Residency In-Training Examination) exam, and had scored above the 95th percentile on Part I of the ABPN.

1

"Maybe that was the beginning of the problem," Dr. Wilson told us later. "My performance on those earlier exams made me complacent."

Other circumstances contributed to this false sense of security. For one thing, Dr. Wilson was employed by a teaching institution—not in a teaching role, to be sure, but doing rapid triage assessments of new outpatients.

"I seemed to be performing well in my job, but I realize now that I had begun to get sloppy. I was taking shortcuts—skimping on the medical history, sometimes omitting the review of systems and family history. Without feedback (no one was really supervising my work), I had begun to view this sort of performance as the norm.

"Then there was my job title: Assistant Professor of Psychiatry at _____ University. I now know that my examiners had no idea where I had trained or where I worked. But I thought that at least they would know I was on the faculty of an excellent training program, and that they would assume I knew my stuff."

Dr. Wilson shifted uneasily and looked embarrassed. "I guess I felt I wanted to impress them with how good I really was. So I spent all of my preparation time listening to Audio Digest tapes and reading journal articles. I was really up on the current literature, but I ignored the basics. I didn't crack a textbook, didn't review old course notes. And, of course, I didn't read DSM-IV."

Mock boards were another point in the preparation that hindered when they should have helped. Although Dr. Wilson had done poorly on mock boards several times during residency, that experience was not sufficient to stimulate a searching mock board before the examination. Instead, a friend who was also a colleague agreed to give half a mock exam, based on a previously recorded videotape. When the videotape could not be located, they instead discussed a patient whom Dr. Wilson knew and could present from memory.

"He said I did fine, but now I know that it was a sketchy, cursory evaluation—a mockery of a mock exam, at best." So the examiner-friend noted no problems, and Dr. Wilson went to the exams blissfully unaware of the disaster that was brewing.

"I didn't feel especially nervous until I met my patient, a woman who obsessed about her husband's pipe smoking. I suddenly realized that I didn't know what questions to ask to diagnose obsessive-compulsive disorder. I panicked. I couldn't think and started to stammer. I glanced at the interviewers—I know you're not supposed to—and one of them seemed to be looking skyward. That glance seemed to say, 'What is this person doing here?' It only added to my terror. There seemed to be no point in going on. All I could focus on was my own anxiety, so I finally stopped the interview before the time was up."

During the question-and-answer session, things went from bad to worse. In retrospect, Dr. Wilson thought that the examiners had even tried to help by suggesting the diagnosis of obsessive-compulsive disorder, but it was to no avail.

"My anxiety level was too great. Without realizing it, I jumped back and forth from Axis I to Axis II. I had forgotten to ask for any developmental history—that's one of the things I don't usually do in my job. But when the examiners asked me if I thought this was an important area to cover, I said 'No!' I thought they were trying to trap me!"

"I didn't need any letter to tell me that I had flunked," Dr. Wilson concluded ruefully. "I knew as soon as I walked out of that examination room. There wasn't a shred of doubt in my mind."

In some cases, of course, the evidence is less clear-cut. But from the stories candidates have told us, it is usually obvious why they failed. And it is fair to say that, although they may not acknowledge it as emphatically as Dr. Wilson did, most candidates who failed come to recognize that it was largely their own behavior, either during the examination or while preparing, that made them Board casualties.

In the final analysis, it is still the examiners' judgment that determines who will pass and who will fail. Even conscientiously applied guidelines—we will discuss them in Chapter 4—cannot completely compensate for the subjectivity inherent in this process. In judging candidates, some examiners use one or more rules of thumb. One is, "Is this a safe physician?" Another is the referral criterion: "Would you refer your own patient to this candidate for treatment?" A "No" answer to either could mean failure.

With a few glaring exceptions (we'll also cover these later on), hardly any single factor will cause a candidate to fail the Boards. Nearly every Board casualty is created by a series of behaviors that in combination yield disaster. They can be divided into two main groups—inadequacies of performance and inadequacies of information—and they are about equally responsible for Part II failures. These two problem areas can come to light nearly anywhere throughout the examination.

Inadequate Performance

Problems Interacting With the Patient

Unsatisfactory interviews unfold in a variety of ways. In the first of these, the candidate fails to develop rapport with the patient. Although it may not be the most important type of error candidates make, to examiners it can be one of the most glaring. Because problems of rapport become evident so early, they can set the tone for the entire exam.

Right from the start, our examiner informants told us, successful candidates

- Orient the patient to the purpose of the exam
- Make introductions all around

- Make the patient feel welcome and appreciated
- Look directly at the patient
- Show empathy, especially for a patient whose story is particularly wrenching

In the words of one examiner, "You rarely see a caring candidate who doesn't do well overall in the examination." Of course, some candidates are kind and even empathic, yet still do not pass. But maneuvers and attitudes that foster good rapport put the candidate way ahead. Unfortunately, perhaps only half the candidates do these things well. When they don't, it is often because severe anxiety has reduced their ability to relate emotionally to their patients. Cultural differences can also inhibit the development of rapport. When patient and candidate come from markedly different backgrounds, they may have trouble understanding one another. Whatever the cause, failure of rapport is not fatal by itself. But it may establish a negative bias in the minds of the examiners. As one examiner put it, "A nonempathic interview is a sign of bad interview technique."

Perhaps to avoid appearing cold or aloof, some candidates go to extremes in the opposite direction. They lean too far forward in their chairs or appear oversolicitous of the patient's comfort. Their expressions of interest seem forced and insincere: "You had to walk all the way to the gas station? Oh, dear, what a *horrible* experience!" This sort of dramatic overempathizing rings false and would set anyone's teeth on edge. Examiners are no exception.

Conduct of the Interview

Winning interviews are all alike in that they get the job done with a minimum of fuss. Losing interviews are of several sorts. Among other problems, there can be too little control, or too much. Or the candidate may neglect to follow up appropriately on what the patient says.

Any of these mistakes can cause trouble, but in our opinion, failure to take charge of the interview is one of the worst because it occurs so often. It may start with the opening question. If that question is vague and nondirective, the patient may conclude that the candidate is only there for a chat. Here is a sample opener from a recent Board casualty: "How's life been treating you?"

Closely related to the vague opening question is what one examiner called "the crime of the directionless interview." Here, the candidate just sits back and absorbs what the patient offers, regardless of its information content. A loquacious patient can easily ramble on for 20 minutes or more, destroying the candidate's chance to obtain the data necessary for a diagnosis. Lack of direction is one of the most serious interviewing errors you can make. If vagueness dominates, it is almost sure to have a lethal effect.

At the other extreme is the overcontrolled interview. This happens when the candidate, perhaps from nervousness, gives the patient no time to tell a story but instead keeps up a barrage of questions throughout the half hour. To a naive observer this candidate might look pretty good: the technique certainly delivers a wealth of information. Unfortunately, it provides insufficient opportunity to learn what is important to the patient.

"It was the reason I had to fail one of the brightest candidates I've ever seen," an examiner recalled. "He knew psychopathology cold, could recite all the diagnostic criteria in the manual. And he could tell me all about any psychotropic agent I could think of. But his interview was terrible! He never made eye contact and didn't seem to care what the patient thought. He just asked one question right after another. By the end, he knew everything about the patient's disease, and very little about the patient."

Other errors in the conduct of the interview have been noted by Napoliello (1977). Among these are awkwardness and inconsistency in the interview structure. The candidate, perhaps spurred on by anxiety, does not conduct a naturally flowing interview, but instead jumps from one subject to another. This process yields less information and more anxiety, and it further reduces control over the interview.

Another behavior that examiners may interpret as lack of control is stopping the interview too abruptly. Instead of a graceful transition from questions to closure ("We only have a minute or so left, so let me ask you this one last question . . ."), the occasional candidate simply stops talking and waits for the patient to be led from the room. Although this lack of common courtesy is deplorable, it is not usually fatal. Still, successful candidates offer their thanks, a handshake, and best wishes to the patients who have helped them with the examination.

Poor Follow-Up on Cues and Clues

Some examinees don't investigate the clues their patients present. This may result from anxiety or from an ill-advised determination to stick with a set interview strategy. Either way, it's a serious error: examiners worry that such candidates lack the observational skills to assess their patients competently. Patients show many behaviors that should serve as cues for further exploration. Which behaviors should be followed up is generally a matter of clinical judgment, but some virtually demand investigation. These include tearfulness, hints about death or suicide, abnormal activity level (either depressed or elevated), and references to substance abuse.

Throughout the interview, you will have to keep alert for situations that require further inquiry. One candidate, interviewing a hypomanic, homosexual man, did not assess the likelihood of AIDS by asking about high-risk sexual acts or the use of condoms. Here is another actual example:

> A woman outpatient with a history of lifelong impulsiveness and personality disorder reported extraordinary anger at her boss, who had fired her the day she was a Board interview patient. The candidate inquired about her feelings, but failed to ask what she planned to do about them. What came to light only after the interview, when the *examiners* began to ask questions, was that she had a gun and planned to kill her former employer as soon as she left the building. In this case, the examiners took the patient literally by the hand and had her admitted to a hospital. The candidate did not fare well.

To be sure, some of these situations are highly unusual, but if they do crop up and you leave them unexplored, you will probably not pass your examination.

Homicidal ideas, thoughts of suicide, depression, substance abuse—these topics are all important to cover in any initial psychiatric interview. Many, though not all, examiners consider them just about indispensable to a passing performance on Part II. However, should you inadvertently leave something out of your interview, you may be able to retrieve the situation later on if, without prompting, you call attention to your omission and show that you recognize how that information is important to the evaluation of your patient.

One examiner recalled that during his own Board examination he had forgotten to ask about drug abuse. He didn't realize his error until he was already well into the presentation of his patient. He immediately admitted the mistake and then quickly outlined what he should have asked and what effect the answers might have had on his recommended diagnosis and treatment. He passed with flying colors.

"You can forget just about anything, and it won't necessarily make you fail," he told us. "But be test-wise: watch the faces of your examiners and pay attention to what they are saying. If an examiner tries to remind you about something— suicidal ideas, for example—and still you don't get it, you're in danger of failing."

High Anxiety

Anxiety is a complicating factor that cuts across the spectrum of candidate performance. Of course, it will exacerbate the problems of any candidate who is doing poorly, but it has also been the downfall of many a well-trained, well-prepared candidate. We know of one psychiatrist whose uncooperative patient so upset him that, when asked after the patient left if he had ever heard of mania, he blurted out, "No!" Another candidate was literally too frightened to utter a single word. For long minutes she struggled to communicate with her examiners, who tried their best to help her. But she finally had to leave the room in defeat. (Studies have shown that women candidates are somewhat more susceptible to the effects of anxiety. But our comments about anxiety and, later, techniques to reduce it apply equally to male and female candidates.)

Less dramatically, but still with a devastating effect on performance, anxiety may cause candidates to behave like automatons. They seldom make eye contact and convey little warmth of affect to their patients. Motor restlessness, a quavering voice, slips of the tongue, and otherwise garbled speech may be other behavioral manifestations of this affective state.

Anxiety has its cognitive effects, too. Some candidates complain of "coming up blank" when asked about material they ordinarily can discuss at length. And examiners often comment that anxiety seems to be at least partly responsible for the rigidity of thinking described earlier. As we shall discuss, anxiety may also precipitate suspiciousness and even hostility toward examiners. This behavior can verge on the pathological.

Nearly every candidate feels some degree of anxiety. According to the estimates of some who have examined for years, about a third of candidates manage to maintain a relatively calm demeanor. Another third appear moderately anxious, but maintain their composure well enough to get through the examination. However, a very considerable minority of candidates are so affected by their own anxiety that their behavior seems pathological. In the words of one examiner, "They're off-scale." They clearly struggle with the form and content of the examination, and although they may ultimately pass, it is only with a supreme effort of will and determination.

Brown (1977) noted that many candidates who fail the Part II exams perform significantly less well due to excessive anxiety. Although we agree that competent performance under stress is ". . . a necessary aspect of the physician's role," it is clear that the stress produced by the exam situation is far greater than you would expect from any ordinary clinical interview. So you should take all reasonable steps to get your own anxiety under control. (We discuss how to deal with anxiety in Chapter 3.)

Personality Clashes

Candidates sometimes report interpersonal problems with their examiners. It is important to note that examiners themselves seldom cite personality clashes as a reason for candidate failure. This may be partly due to the checks-and-balances nature of the multiple-examiner system. With two primary examiners, a floating examiner, and an ABPN director all involved in the grading process, there is always someone who will say, "Let's ignore the personality clash—that's not what's important." Nonetheless, from time to time, candidates do have interpersonal difficulties with their examiners, who, being human, are as susceptible to irritation as anyone else. But keep in mind that when examiners do become irritated, it is usually in response to nonprofessional or inappropriate behavior on the part of a candidate. The following are just a few examples.

Making wisecracks, especially about the patient, is a sure-fire way to alienate examiners. Arguing is another. "It's stupid to argue," exclaimed one examiner, who assured us that a real confrontation is almost sure to work against any candidate. But the stress of the moment may adversely affect the judgment, and ultimately the candidacy, of even the most competent candidate.

> "Bad vibes" did in Dr. Alice Baker, who thought she detected instant dislike in the tone of her examiner. "That examiner was a woman, too," Dr. Baker said later, while she was studying for her repeat Part II examination. "I somehow got it into my head that she disliked me because she didn't want competition from another female. I thought it was bad vibes, right from the start. She seemed to be attacking my diagnosis, and it made me angry. I thought that I had to maintain my principles, so I fought back. I was really sorry I had argued when the notice of failure arrived in the mail."

When candidates break off the interview with time to spare, examiners worry that the time has not been fully used to obtain all the relevant information. Some examiners interpret this behavior as lack of rapport, though some also see it as arrogance. One examiner told us: "These candidates seem to be saying that they can do what no one else can—a really complete psychiatric examination in 20 minutes. If you do finish a little early, I don't want to see you just sit around and wait for the patient to leave. You can always ask more questions. And I don't mean, 'Is there anything else you would like to tell me?' Of course there isn't! What the patient really wants is to go back to the ward and have lunch. The sort of question I expect is, 'Now I'd like to hear some more about your family.' Or any other area that hasn't been explored fully. And there'll be dozens."

Candidates may also appear arrogant if they present themselves as experts in some area. Such an attitude can have an unfortunate effect on the perceptions of the examiners, even when the candidate does have some extraordinary qualifications. One such candidate fixated on lupus erythematosus as a principal diagnosis and maintained that position throughout the question-and-answer session. The examiners regarded this as "an odd tangent." Another candidate insisted on doing a neurological examination—but left out the mental status exam!

Gaming the System

Some candidates try to figure out what responses will please the examiners. In so doing, they give the appearance of trying to play the game rather than demonstrating their ability to take care of patients. Often, they come to grief.

> Dr. Ben Carver recommended a tricyclic antidepressant for a severely depressed patient. The examiner thought that was fine and then asked about psychotherapy. Dr. Carver agreed, and, because he thought the examiner looked like an analyst, said he would see the patient in psychotherapy three times a week. The candidate wasn't an analyst himself, so he was rather stuck for an answer when asked what use he would make of those sessions. He stammered out something about working on "separation-individuation issues," but later admitted that he was "just BS-ing."
>
> "I was dishonest. I thought both examiners were analysts, and that I was telling them what they would want to hear," he commented. Later, while preparing to repeat his Part II examination, he pointed out that it would have been better to concentrate on what he knew about firsthand. "I could have referred the patient for more intensive management, if I'd honestly thought it was necessary," he said.

Inadequate Information

During the second half of your exam, you will interact with the examiners on a number of different issues. These include a presentation of the patient, diagnosis, and recommendations for management. In each of these, it is important to demonstrate skill and care that will persuade your examiners that you are a competent specialist.

The Presentation

Because it demonstrates how well you have understood your patient, the presentation is critically important to your performance. Unfortunately, many candidates have difficulty with this seemingly elementary exercise, which is so familiar even to third-year medical students.

At the root of the problem is an inability to organize the data. Many candidates seem unable to digest the information and report it in a fashion that is both coherent and interesting. Instead, they regurgitate the unprocessed history pretty much as it came from the patient. Some carry this to the illogical extreme and simply read the notes they have made! The examiners, who want more than an unedited instant replay, interrupt to ask questions. They are dissatisfied, the candidate is flustered, and the presentation is off to a bad start.

Trouble in the Differential

The differential diagnosis is another source of grief; most candidates seem to have some trouble here. Examiners are quick to point out that usually it isn't a matter of "the wrong diagnosis"—the rightness or wrongness of diagnosis isn't what Part II is all about. What examiners want to find is a pattern of sound diagnostic thinking that will serve well for future patients. Examiners cite two sorts of diagnostic error:

1. Candidates cannot defend diagnoses intellectually. When asked to state their diagnostic criteria, they stumble. Worse, some will try to wing it, making up criteria as they go along. Examiners easily recognize the deception. They feel more comfortable with candidates who recognize and acknowledge their deficiencies than they do with candidates who bluff and stonewall.
2. Some candidates become so fixated on one diagnosis that they will not consider alternatives. The diagnosis may be implausible:

   A 35-year-old man with chronic delusions and auditory hallucinations was diagnosed as having temporal lobe epilepsy on the basis of an old head injury and the report of "odd smells." The candidate would not be budged from this diagnosis.

Even if the diagnosis is plausible, the candidate who is unwilling to consider other possibilities may seem uncomfortably inflexible:

One extremely well trained academic psychiatrist was assigned to interview a patient who showed the classic manic symptoms of push of speech, flight of ideas, and hyperactivity.

"What other diagnoses would you consider in your differential?" asked the examiner.

"None," replied the candidate. "This patient is in the manic phase of bipolar affective disorder."

Despite repeated questioning and ample opportunity to suggest other conditions one should consider in a patient with manic behavior, the candidate stuck to his guns—and died there, unwilling even to discuss a clinical differential.

Candidates sometimes won't give a favorite or most likely diagnosis, even when strongly pressured by their examiners to do so. "It drives us all batty," said one examiner. "Maybe they're afraid we're going to trick them, but all we really want is a diagnosis to discuss with them. It could be anything, as long they can support it with data. But when candidates absolutely refuse to choose a diagnosis, I can't even evaluate their clinical judgment."

Similar problems show up on the videotape examination, where adequate data may be lacking.

"They're not being tested on the diagnosis," another examiner stated, "but on their ability to think through a clinical problem. What we want is candidates to think out loud and show us how they would reason through a clinical problem. They should consider the data that fit and recognize those that don't fit. Some candidates diagnose schizophrenia no matter what. Others overinterpret the data and make definite diagnoses they can't defend. Instead, they should talk about the questions they'd like to ask, the tests they'd run on this patient. If they feel uncomfortable making a definitive diagnosis, they should say something like this: 'Most likely this is a case of _____ because of _____. But one piece of data that doesn't fit is _____. I'd want to know more about _____.' "

Poor Planning

Even with an adequate interview and differential diagnosis, candidates may recommend management and treatment that seem unwise. Some can't reason through a plan for further evaluation. A classic example would be ordering an evaluation with the Wechsler Adult Intelligence Scale, but not being able to state what help to expect from it. When the dexamethasone suppression test (DST) was at its height of popularity, candidates failed to understand it in two ways: how to administer it and how to interpret it. According to examiners, some candidates appeared to believe that the DST was a definitive test for depression, rather than a device that can sometimes augment the clinical history and mental status exam.

Treatment Failures

In recent years, most candidates have been quite well versed in psychopharmacology. Once-common errors such as recommending insufficient doses of tricyclic antidepressants are now unusual. Not knowing pharmacotherapy complications such as the neuroleptic malignant syndrome continues to be a problem for some, however. The consequences may be particularly dire when it is the candidate who has suggested the drug in the first place.

When asked to recommend treatment for a depressed young married man, Dr. Kim Larson suggested trazodone "because it has fewer anticholinergic side effects." The following exchange then took place:

EXAMINER. What side effects would you expect?
DR. LARSON. Well, drowsiness. But I'd give it all at night. He's been having
       trouble sleeping, anyway.
EXAMINER. Anything else?
DR. LARSON. Not that I can think of.
EXAMINER. Does the fact that he's male influence your thinking any?
DR. LARSON. No.

After the examination had been completed, the examiners had a heated discussion about this performance. One even argued in favor of failure, not because Dr. Larson appeared unaware that priapism was one of trazodone's potential side effects, but because the side effect was serious and concerned a drug the candidate had suggested.

We hasten to point out that few of the examiners we interviewed would fail an otherwise satisfactory candidate on the basis of this one error. However, it was also their consensus that a single serious error could (though rarely) cause failure. Such a cataclysmic mistake would probably be one that, if put into practice, might kill someone. Here are a few examples of mistakes that could be fatal both to your patient and to your candidacy:

- Prescribing a monoamine oxidase inhibitor without a low-tyramine diet
- Recommending a massive dose of medication (e.g., 10 g of lithium per day)
- Giving a month's supply of amitriptyline to a suicidal patient
- Failing to recognize a major complication such as the central cholinergic syndrome

Although examiners don't all agree on this point, we talked with some who would fail a candidate for committing any one of several errors not related to drugs:

- Not investigating suicidal ideas in a patient who has demonstrated predictors of suicide such as depression, alcoholism, or borderline personality structure
- Not asking a patient with a history of violence about homicidal ideas
- Not asking about the use of drugs or alcohol
- Throughout the exam, never making eye contact with the patient

Examiners regard with suspicion *any* candidate who does not ask *any* patient about substance abuse, mood disorder, and ideas of suicide, but most would probably not take such a hard-line approach as to recommend automatic failure for one of these omissions. However, major errors like these do make it much more difficult to justify passing an examinee, especially one whose candidacy is already on shaky footing. Above nearly everything else, your examiners must believe that you are a clinician who will deliver safe care.

Rather than a lack of knowledge about pharmacotherapy, the recent tendency among failing candidates has been to understand little else. One examiner told us that he favors candidates who start with a "wide-angle view of the therapeutic spectrum." Other examiners might express it a bit differently: examinees are evaluated on their ability to consider psychosocial, behavioral, psychotherapeutic, and biological approaches to psychiatric illness (the biopsychosocial model). This wide-angle evaluation also focuses on practical questions such as whether or not to hospitalize. Consider this example of one candidate whose focus was too narrow:

The patient had schizophrenia and had been hospitalized for the fourth time.

EXAMINER. What treatment would you recommend for this patient?
CANDIDATE. Neuroleptics.
EXAMINER. But this patient has been consistently refusing medications.
CANDIDATE. Well, I'd give him depot neuroleptics.
EXAMINER. What about his lifelong problem dealing with authority figures?
CANDIDATE. Only neuroleptics will help him very much.

Later this examiner said: "The candidate failed for recommending nothing but drug treatment for an obviously refractory patient. He didn't have to be an analyst, but he did have to know that this problem can be approached in various ways. And candidates won't pass if they don't recognize that noncompliance with medications is a problem that should be approached with something other than more drug therapy."

Dealing With the Difficult Patient

Admittedly, it is hard to know how to proceed with some patients. Difficult problems such as personality disorder, anorexia nervosa, gender identity disorders, and somatization disorder offer no easy cookbook approach. When confronted with one of these situations, candidates will sometimes stumble, perhaps because of the amorphous nature of the problem or perhaps because there is no single adequate solution.

For a difficult patient, as with any other patient, examiners emphasize the importance of approaching therapy with a framework in mind. Citing the example of a histrionic patient who abused drugs, one said, "There probably isn't a single, good treatment for a patient like this one. But one candidate I examined tried to create one by picking up on the elements of a depressive disorder and recommending tricyclic antidepressants. What I'd hoped to hear was some consideration of the possible etiologies of this condition. It might have prompted the candidate to suggest psychosocial management rather than attempts at biological treatment, but I got none of this."

Other Problems

Candidates can present a variety of other problems during the question-and-answer session.

- Some candidates present factual material well enough, but cannot describe feelings. They have trouble interpreting affect and may themselves show little feeling for the emotional state of the patient.
- Candidates who try to fill up the entire half hour with the presentation of the patient may give the appearance of trying to avoid answering questions.
- Candidates sometimes fail to use criteria to defend a favorite diagnosis. Instead of listing some of the DSM-IV criteria for schizophrenia, one candidate insisted on that diagnosis solely because "the patient has had a long history of hallucinations." Examiners emphasize that it is not necessary to know cold every criterion for every diagnosis. But to pass, candidates must have a working knowledge of the basis for diagnosis in modern psychiatry.
- Candidates sometimes introduce topics they are ill prepared to discuss (see the case of Dr. Kim Larson, cited earlier in this chapter).
- Similarly, technical terms are sometimes introduced by candidates who cannot define them accurately.

But candidates do *not* fail because they cannot answer questions concerning minutiae. As Maleson et al. (1980) note, "Difficulties in discussion of fundamental issues are a much greater source of failure than the feared questions about psychiatric obscurities." They also state that, whereas most candidates come well prepared for discussions of psychopharmacology, many "do not seem geared to apply such familiar topics as psychodynamics, principles and problems of psychotherapy, and hospital management to their patients." They suggest that "it is possible that these matters are harder to talk about, particularly for those who are not very articulate." (All quotations from p. 839.)

Summing Up

When candidates fail, it is almost invariably because they have violated some basic rule of the practice of medicine or some principle of conduct between human beings. This is cause for optimism, inasmuch as medicine can be learned and behavior can be modified. Candidates can learn to control most of these behaviors. That is what the following chapters are all about.

Chapter 2 ————————————————

Preparing for Part II

Applying for the Boards

When Should You Take the Boards?

For most, this brief section comes too late. If you're already a candidate, you can't control how long it has been since residency. But on the chance that you have not yet taken Part I of the ABPN, or if you have taken it and you're debating whether (or when) to go ahead with Part II, then our advice is: Do it now!

Once you have passed Part I, you have 6 years (or three tries, whichever comes first) to pass Part II before you have to start all over again. But there is no advantage to putting off Part II. Here is a partial list of reasons:

- Many Board candidates are fresh from their training programs. Like it or not, their level of information raises examiners' expectations for all candidates.
- You'll have better retention of the didactic material soon after you have learned it.
- If you haven't moved too far away, your contacts at your training program will be fresher should you want help with preparation.
- The longer it has been since you completed training, the more opportunity there is for bad habits to creep into your routine of doing an initial interview.
- There's something to be said for the group support you get when sharing the experience with friends.

We don't mean that you're automatically in for a bad time if you finished your residency a number of years ago. You might need more time to review the didactic material, and the mock board exam (discussed later in this chapter) is more important than ever, if such a thing is possible. Some older candidates have complained of the discomfort of being interviewed by examiners who are years younger than they are. But the increase in assurance and patient skills that come from years of psychiatric practice may partly compensate for these drawbacks.

Get Your Application In

Boards are given several times each year at various locations throughout the country. In recent years, the exams have been held in midwinter, spring, and late fall in three different cities, representing the East Coast, the West Coast, and the Midwest. The ABPN currently tries to assign first-time candidates to an examination site close to home. Unfortunately, this is not always possible, and some candidates may still find themselves flying hundreds of miles (or more). Repeat candidates are assigned on a space-available basis and are less likely to be given a nearby exam site.

Taking the exam locally has obvious advantages. Of course, you avoid the expense and fatigue of prolonged air travel and the disorientation and physical discomfort that some people suffer with jet lag. A less obvious benefit is that by staying close to home you may also avoid unfamiliar customs, dialects, and medical facilities that could lessen rapport and generate diagnostic confusion. The moral seems clear: Apply early. It will help you to get an examination site close to home, of course, but there is another benefit for the early bird. Having the registration receipt in hand may stimulate you to get busy with your program of study.

While you are at it, you might as well make airline and hotel reservations, too, if you need them. Unless the exam site is just across town, we'd strongly advise you to get a hotel room the night before the exam. There's so much tension associated with the exam itself that it seems pointless bravado to add the frustration of freeway driving and city traffic to the day's angst.

The question of where to stay can present a problem. For obvious reasons, the principal hotel is invariably large and usually has a room rate to match. If you can, avoid the temptation to stay at the EconoRest down the street. The extra money you spend for the night (rarely, two nights) at the Ritz may not guarantee you a better night's sleep, but it can limit the running around you have to do on examination day.

Mock Boards

You'd never even consider taking a written examination such as Part I of the ABPN without preparation. For an oral exam, there are all the same reasons to study, plus one more: if you make a mistake, it's hard to erase. Whereas your residency program probably trained you to be an excellent psychiatrist, it may have prepared you less well to be an excellent Part II candidate. The time to find out is not during the exam, but months before.

What Is a Mock Board?

Mock boards are a lot like mock turtle soup: a bit of a sham, but close enough to give you a taste of the real thing. A mock board examination can accomplish two things: it can tell you how well prepared you are, and it can serve as a tension-reducing rehearsal.

Everything about a mock board examination should be as close to the real thing as you can manage. You should spend a half-hour interviewing a patient you have never met before in the presence of at least one psychiatrist examiner. The examiner, who should be thoroughly familiar with the Board examination goals and procedures, should then proceed to question you about the interview and the deductions you make from it. At the conclusion, you should receive a critique about your performance in all the areas that will be evaluated in the real thing.

Candidates who have been through this sort of rehearsal invariably report that the dry run lessens their anticipatory anxiety. But the greater benefit of the mock board examination is not therapeutic; it is diagnostic. Think of it as a checkup to make sure the following skills are all healthy:

- Interviewing (including information gathering and personal interaction)
- Diagnosis
- Therapeutics
- Summarizing information
- Making a logical formulation

We really cannot emphasize strongly enough how much we recommend this initial diagnostic examination, but with the following two rules we'd like to try:

Rule 1. Take a mock board examination

- Even if you just graduated from residency (some programs underemphasize interviewing and diagnostic skills)

- Even if you're the busiest psychiatrist in six counties (you'll use your study time more efficiently if you pinpoint your weaknesses early)
- Even if this is the very material you teach to residents (remember the saying that the physician who attempts self-diagnosis has a fool for a doctor and a fool for a patient)

Rule 2. On the off chance that you still decide not to take a diagnostic exam, see Rule 1.

Selecting a Mock Board Examiner

By now you should have the idea that we believe a mock board exam is a *must* for every Part II candidate. But don't just walk down the hall and ask for help from the colleague you happened to have lunch with last Thursday. For something that is as important to you as the Boards, you want the best professional help you can get.

Of course, you should select someone who has already passed the exam. Preferably, it should be someone who has taught enough to have witnessed a wide variety of interviewing styles, both good and bad. You also want someone you don't know too well, who will feel free to offer criticism where you need it. After all, you want useful pointers on your performance, not just praise for your personality.

Beware the Inexperienced Examiner

Try to find someone who participated in the Boards as an examiner—recently, if at all possible, so as to be knowledgeable about the current procedures and rules for grading. Having an insider's view may also prevent your mock board examiner from burdening you with bad advice. Trying to be helpful, one mock examiner we know of advised, "Don't ask the patient what he's been told about his diagnosis." Another offered, "Never open your interview by asking the patient why he came into therapy." Both of these gems were apparently based on misguided notions of what was fair in an examination situation. Neither advisor had any experience as a board examiner. Both candidates took the advice, to their sorrow.

Using the Criticisms

The criticisms your mock examiner makes could help you decide how much time to devote to preparation and how to apportion it. If your problems seem to be largely academic, you will want to spend more time studying the books mentioned later in this chapter and in the reading list in Appendix E. Problems with interview skills should send you to the relevant chapters in this book (Chapters 5–8) and in other volumes dealing with the psychiatric interview. Problems with the interview should also be a signal for you to practice on your own with another dozen or so patients. You may be able to "borrow" patients from a local university, state, or Veterans hospital for this purpose. Stick to the half-hour format, and review your performance to see how much information you were able to get from each interview.

Any significant criticism the mock examiner makes of your physician-patient relationship should give you pause. For a fully trained psychiatrist this is a serious criticism indeed, one that should be carefully evaluated. You would naturally like to conclude that the criticism only reflects an interpersonal problem between you and that particular examiner. This thought is comforting, but don't succumb to it. What you need is not solace, but a second opinion. Find another teacher-examiner (again, someone you don't know too well) and take a second diagnostic mock board. Tell your second examiner what happened the first time, and ask for particularly close criticism of the interpersonal aspects of your patient interview.

If the second opinion is quite different from the first, you should sit down with each of the examiners and try to determine where the problem lies. If certain types of patients give you trouble, you should try several practice sessions with just these types. On the other hand, you may learn that you are inordinately sensitive to certain types of exam questions (or examiners!). You should approach this sort of problem by analyzing the questions (or personalities) and follow up with several sessions of cognitive rehearsal.

If the second opinion is no different from the first, you may need intensive remediation, which is beyond the scope of this book. At minimum, you should plan to take a Board examination review course, like those we mention later on in this chapter.

Practice, Practice

Regardless of the reason, if you did not do well on your first mock board examination, you should try a number of timed practice interviews by yourself. With the patient's permission, tape-record some of them for later analysis—you may learn how you could phrase questions better or respond more quickly to cues from the patient. Also use this time to practice formulating questions clearly and succinctly so that you can obtain the most precise information in the least time possible. After each practice session, review the tape to see how much information you managed to collect in 30 minutes. You may want to augment these practice sessions with mini mock boards conducted by colleagues—perhaps other psychiatrists practicing for the same examination.

For your practice interviews, try to choose patients with a wide spectrum of diagnoses and personal backgrounds. This may be especially important if you are in private practice, perhaps specializing in psychotherapy, and you don't often encounter patients who have psychoses, suicidal depressions, substance abuse, or severe character pathology. These are exactly the types of patient most likely to turn up on the exam. In any event, venturing outside your normal sphere of practice should repay you by honing both your diagnostic acumen and your interpersonal skills on a variety of patient types.

Some candidates found it helpful to prepare a short speech on several of the areas they believed that they were likely to be questioned about. This stratagem may be justified if you worry about being incapacitated by stage fright. If this is the case, you might want to outline brief presentations on the diagnosis, etiology, and management of commonly encountered disorders such as schizophrenia, mood disorder, borderline personality disorder, substance-related disorders, and dementia. Then, should you suddenly go blank, you can fall back on automatic pilot and coast for a few moments until you recover. But be warned that if what you say is not strictly appropriate to the patient under discussion, your examiners may feel put off by canned speech that represents what you know, not how you would apply it in practice. So be careful how you use a prepared speech; if used at all, it may be most appropriate during the discussion of the videotape.

If you have taken some of these steps because of problems identified on an earlier mock board, arrange to take another mock board several weeks before the actual examination. It should provide a useful check on the progress you have made since you began studying and help you identify any remaining problems with your interview technique or presentation. And the experience of yet another practice session should validate your efforts and give you the extra confidence you need.

We should add that we don't think it's possible to over-practice for the Boards. The twin advantages of experiencing more patients and reducing your anxiety make more, rather than fewer, mock board exams the ideal. Some academic psychiatrists report that candidates from their institutions now average three or four mock boards before embarking on the real thing.

Book Learning

Of course, you will want to put in a significant amount of time reading, both to bone up on the basics of psychiatry and to review what has been written about interviewing. You should review a good textbook of general psychiatry. You may not want to read the entire multivolume set of the original, but the current edition of *Kaplan and Sadock's Synopsis of Psychiatry: Behavioral Sciences, Clinical Psychiatry* by Harold I. Kaplan, Benjamin J. Sadock, and Jack A. Grebb (the 1994 edition is the 7th) provides a good, succinct overview that can be read in digestible, chapter-long chunks. Another recent, excellent general reference work is *The American Psychiatric Press Textbook of Psychiatry,* Second Edition, edited by Robert E. Hales, Stuart C. Yudofsky, and John A. Talbott (1994). A number of other good texts are on the American market, any of which should suffice as a reference for your questions about general psychiatry.

To be most helpful, the text you select should be keyed to DSM-IV (American Psychiatric Association 1994). This volume is described in ABPN literature as the primary authority on psychiatric diagnostic nomenclature. All clinicians can relate to it because it does a good job of remaining, as advertised, largely atheoretical. It provides a common basis for discussion of mental disorders, so every candidate should be thoroughly familiar with it. You shouldn't try to memorize this document (though some candidates have done just that), but you should know the principles that sparked its construction and underlie its diagnostic schemes. Also, several diagnostic categories are likely to come up for discussion during your examination. You should review the criteria for these often enough so that you know them well. They include principally the diagnoses listed in Table 9–1 (Chapter 9). In addition, you should be familiar with the criteria for schizophreniform psychosis, schizoaffective disorder, and any other diagnoses about which you feel uncertain.

But there is no specific textbook for the Boards. You have already passed Part I, and should therefore have a good working knowledge of the clinical and theoretical material that can be learned from the printed page. If, after you have read *Boarding Time,* DSM-IV, and an up-to-date general psychiatry text, you still feel the need for more reading, you might consult any of the specialty volumes we list in Appendix E. We have often suggested reading material to our friends, but our endorsement doesn't mean that these books are necessary, and certainly not sufficient, to pass the Boards. The books we recommend are simply those we favor.

Time Spent

How much time should you plan to spend on reading, practice interviewing, and other activities before taking the examination? The answer depends heavily on your anxiety level, your sense of preparedness, the outcome of your first mock board examination, and whether you are a first-time candidate. It is theoretically possible for a well-trained candidate to take and pass the oral exam with little preparation other than frequently evaluating psychiatric patients, as would be done in a private practice or teaching position.

Few candidates have that much confidence in their training; most will want to augment it with additional preparation. One survey (Brown 1977) found that the average candidate studied 4 or 5 hours a week for 4–6 months. To capitalize on short-term retention, it was common to double the amount of time spent in the 2 weeks or so immediately preceding the exam. Although there have been no subsequent surveys, talking with recent candidates leads us to believe that this pattern has not changed appreciably. However, this amount of time (120 hours, exclusive of time spent studying for Part I) is probably more than most candidates actually need. You will use your time more efficiently if you take your mock exam first and use it as a guide for outlining your course of study.

Proprietary Courses

Over the years, Board review courses have been offered by various institutions and individuals. Although the promotions for these courses are often aimed at all candidates, repeating candidates are overrepresented among those who enroll. (However, one unusually cautious candidate attended three such courses before successfully completing the exam—on his first try!) The courses are of three basic types:

1. Those that present factually oriented material in lecture format, more appropriate for Part I
2. Those that emphasize method and style in a variety of presentations, better for Part II
3. Those that combine the above approaches, which are probably the best of all

Some courses have been organized by psychiatric societies, others by departments of psychiatry at universities. Still others are proprietary, organized on a for-profit basis by individuals who may offer Board review courses in a number of medical specialties. Because the quality of Board review courses can be quite variable and their cost is usually high, you should investigate carefully before choosing.

Any review course that promises real help for the Part II candidate should include a session during which a faculty member individually evaluates your interview technique with actual patients. Each class participant should have the opportunity to star in at least one such mock board drill. We discourage Part II candidates from relying exclusively on any course that does not feature these individual assessment sessions.

As a sort of standard, we will describe one university-sponsored course. This course lasted from Friday evening through Sunday afternoon (an extra half-day course on anxiety reduction was also offered—for an additional fee). The instruction began with a lecture and demonstration, during which a junior faculty member acted the part of a candidate taking a Board examination. An actual psychiatric patient added to the feeling that this was the real thing. The mock candidate was subsequently questioned by an examiner, just as would be the case for a genuine Part II examination.

Active participation began on Saturday morning and continued through Sunday afternoon for a total of 8 hours on each weekend day. Divided into groups of six, each participant took a mock board examination on each of the 2 days. The candidates had the added benefit of a different examiner each time. Each mock board was witnessed by the other five members of the group, so that by the end of the weekend each participant had experienced a total of 12 mock board examinations. (Most also took advantage of a 3-hour Saturday evening opportunity to examine more patients, with fellow candidates taking the role of examiner.) This course also presented two videotapes of patients, followed by discussion in small groups, and two lectures, one on the changes that have been incorporated into DSM and one on how to present a formulation.

Even though it was only practice, participants found the mock boards nearly as anxiety provoking as the actual examination. (One candidate even reported some trouble sleeping the weekend of the course.) This extremely intensive course was praised by the participants, both for its content and for its desensitization of the candidates to the stress. They reported that the desensitization later generalized to the ABPN.

Chapter 3 ───────────────────

Presenting Yourself for the Exam

Over the years, life has become easier for ABPN candidates. Now they have only 2 hours of oral examination, not 6 hours as was the case when the Boards were first given. Today's candidates no longer face the prospect of examining a neurology patient, as was the case even in the 1970s. Even the burdens of travel have been eased by the recent change in ABPN policy that preferentially assigns first-time candidates to the exam site closest to home.

Getting There

Once you have passed Part I of the Boards, you will be automatically assigned to a Part II examination time and site. You must pay the fee ($725 as of this writing, though it is scheduled to increase in 1995) by the deadline specified in the letter that notifies you of your exam site assignment, or you will be dropped from the rolls for that examination date and site. Should this happen, you risk being assigned later to an exam site farther from home. Moral: After receiving your packet of information from the ABPN, send back the registration form along with your check as soon as you can. If you change your mind, you can still cancel up to 90 days before the exam and receive a full refund. After that, you would forfeit the entire fee and have to start again.[1]

If you do have to travel across time zones, you should take what steps you can to be sure you are in the best possible physical shape for the examination. To reduce the effects of jet lag, several days before you fly start getting up and going to bed at an hour that accords with the time demands of the exam schedule and the time zone of your host city. Try to schedule a direct (preferably nonstop) flight. Eat lightly but regularly, and don't drink alcohol on the flight. You should also plan not to go out drinking with old buddies the night before the exam. (Some candidates have enjoyed their reunions so thoroughly that they themselves couldn't have subtracted serial 7s the following day!)

The point is that you want to feel sharp from that moment on the day before the exam when you hear the introductory remarks by the Executive Secretary of the ABPN. Then, prepare to note the last-minute schedule changes and any useful bits of advice. Take it to heart when you hear that the Board and its examiners want you to pass and will not try to trick you. They mean it.

For supper the evening before, eat lightly and normally. Again, don't drink alcohol. If you feel you must study, limit yourself to an hour or so and then relax with television or a dull book.

On the morning of the big day, be sure to arise in plenty of time. After your months of careful preparation, there's no point in setting yourself up for unnecessary anxiety by oversleeping. So set your alarm *and* leave a wake-up call with the hotel operator. You may sleep better if you protect yourself with the "belt and suspenders" approach to early rising.

Dress for Success

Examiners are human. Despite their best intentions to focus on the interview, they may be influenced by a candidate's hygiene and dress. When you think about it, this isn't especially outrageous. Part of your success as a psychiatrist—the patient's willingness to divulge information and to follow your instructions—is pegged to your image as a professional person. It should come as no great surprise that your examiners might judge your competence by the same criteria a patient would use.

Although we would agree that image isn't everything, it is *something*. In a

---

1 If you have specific questions about times, sites, fees, or other conditions of the Part II examinations, write to the ABPN at 500 Lake Cook Road, Suite 335, Deerfield, IL 60015. For the answer to a question that cannot wait for the mail, you can telephone (708) 945-7900 and ask for the Part II Coordinator. In our experience, the people in this office are well informed and cheerfully helpful.

one-shot interview, it takes on added importance. You'll feel better and you may perform better if you stand tall, act competent, and dress the part.

Of course, some rules are nothing but pure social convention. Steffi Graf could undoubtedly play championship tennis in a T-shirt and cutoffs, but the officials at Wimbledon wouldn't let her on the court. What physicians wear is also a matter of convention. Most of us could practice equally good psychiatry wearing three-piece suits or scuba-diving gear. But with all the other uncertainties inherent in the exam process, it would be foolish to attract unfavorable attention with clothing that some examiners might consider unprofessional.

Most examiners will have a fairly high tolerance for individuality of clothing style. But note that secular trends in dress do change with time. Whereas long hair and sandals (for men) might have been acceptable in the 1970s, today they might raise eyebrows. Many examiners might think that a candidate who dresses that way is more eager to make a personal statement than to practice psychiatry. (We continue to wonder how it worked out for one candidate who appeared for the exam in bib overalls.)

Aim for a professionally appropriate style of dress. This means a suit and tie for men and a suit, nice dress, or skirt, blouse, and jacket for women. The general rule is "If it is inappropriate for your office, it is inappropriate for the Boards." After all, you don't want to wear anything that might deflect the focus from your abilities as a psychiatrist.

You might want to put a fresh (but opened) package of facial tissues into your pocket or purse. You can't be sure that the host facility will have them available, and you never know in advance who in the exam room may need one.

Dealing With Anxiety

Nearly all candidates are anxious. (Candidates report that even *reading* about the Boards, as in the first edition of this book, is anxiety provoking!) You don't have to spend much time at any Board exam to see the effects: dozens of physicians milling around, pacing, and laughing nervously. If you happen to have the nerves of a cat burglar, you can probably skip the rest of this section. But if you don't enjoy the prospect of working the high wire without a net, read on.

Defining Anxiety

Anxiety is generally recognized as having three components:

- *Physiological.* You have dry mouth; your heart races and skips beats; you feel tremulous, sweaty, and light-headed.

- *Behavioral.* Your hands shake. Your dry mouth makes it difficult to talk. When you do, your speech seems stilted. Your movements are stereotyped. The overall quality of your performance decreases.
- *Subjective.* You become aware of the physiological changes going on. You have trouble concentrating on the matters at hand. You feel a sense of impending doom and you may want to run.

These signs and symptoms are influenced by a number of factors that include sleep, exercise, and the use of substances such as caffeine, alcohol, and tobacco. But your experience of anxiety will probably be most strongly colored by your other emotions, which will in turn be largely determined by your expectations about the exam process. Of course, attitudes vary widely. Especially before the examination, many candidates may take a somewhat jaundiced view of the proceedings. But by the time it's all over, most candidates view the process as a positive one and regard the ABPN staff as courteous, efficient, and helpful.

Reducing Your Anxiety

For the anxiety you may feel during your Board examination, thorough preparation beats any treatment. We have already discussed some of the steps you can take to prepare (see Chapter 2):

- Taking mock board exams
- Attending Board review courses
- Preparing outlines of diagnostic areas that have been a problem for you

To those steps we might add other techniques you already know about that may prove helpful:

- Trying biofeedback
- Using behavior modification
- Imaging success

A source of anxiety that sometimes arises during the examination itself is lack of feedback from the examiners. One perennial complaint of candidates is the anxiety-enhancing effect of the examiners' affects during the interrogation sessions. "All I got was the 'blank screen' approach" and "You'd think I was on the couch instead of taking the exam" are typical comments.

It is true that your examiners won't give you the sort of feedback and reassurance that would reduce your anxiety. But their behavior is not an indication of hostility. Most examiners have a great deal of empathy for the candidates they examine; many admit that the anxiety of their examinees often causes *them* considerable anxiety, too. Some have bemoaned the difficulty of having any pleasant interaction in a situation where all personal topics are forbidden and most candidates are anxious.

As we explain in Chapter 4, examiners are asked to show neither approval nor disapproval, but rather to present a facade of friendly neutrality. Your examiners' goal in maintaining expressionless faces is to avoid signals that could either suggest answers or steer you in the wrong direction. Of course, the method has its failures. Quick and Robinowitz (1981) cite one dismayed candidate who reported leaving the oral exam with the feeling she had failed, despite the fact that she was one of the best candidates of that exam session. Many examiners have told us how they have wanted, when encountering a forlorn-looking candidate who has just passed, to give a pat of approval and say, "It's okay. Enjoy the rest of the day." But even that amount of human contact is disallowed, because in this circumstance an examiner could not know whether or not the candidate had passed the *other* half of Part II.

If you feel that an examiner is giving you the blank screen stare, there are several tactics you can use. But first, here's one you shouldn't use: Don't call the examiner on this issue! You won't improve the situation any, and you certainly won't improve the examiner's affect toward you by pointing out that the ABPN requests that examiners interact pleasantly.

Instead, remind yourself in advance that one or both examiners might not show much affect. If that turns out to be the case, try to ignore this behavior as best you can. Use your interpersonal skills and concentrate on relating to the patient or, during the question-and-answer session, to the other examiner. If it helps, try regarding this interaction as you would regard one with a patient who cannot express emotion normally: it is the patient who has the problem, not you!

Drugs to Combat Anxiety?

You probably tell your patients what we tell ours: avoid using medication if you possibly can. But the Board examination is a situation that may tempt you to test the limits of that rule. If you are exceptionally anxiety prone, medication may prove vital. However, an examiner tells of one candidate who carried self-medication too far.

> This candidate started out looking pretty good in the first exam (it was the era of several exams in one day), but by midmorning his speech was slurred and by noon he was staggering. It turned out that for courage he had been nipping at a hip flask throughout the morning. We finally had to put him to bed!

A more recent exam session occasioned a similar unfortunate incident. Without a doubt, alcohol is out as the drug of choice.

So which ones should you consider? Because of possible side effects of drowsiness, depression, and decreased performance, we don't recommend benzodiazepines. (Of course, if you are already taking one of these drugs on a regular basis, the Board exam is no time to stop.) But a beta-adrenergic receptor–blocking agent such as propranolol may help a lot.

Double-blind studies have shown that small doses of propranolol taken before a stress-inducing stimulus can reduce the physiological effects of anxiety. Tachycardia is decreased, and dry mouth is less bothersome. Objective ratings of performance improve, too, as do subjective feelings of well-being. In short, this drug may reduce anticipatory anxiety and help you perform better. One candidate who was repeating the Boards described its effects as "unbelievably helpful."

The usual dose is 20–40 mg taken 60–90 minutes before the exam. But don't wait until that day to try it for the first time. If you are one of those for whom the drug has negative effects on memory and performance, you'll want to find that out when you have less at stake. If you decide you are one of the exceptional candidates who should try it, do so before one of your mock board exams.

Warning

The ABPN is quite clear: it wants to examine only physicians who are unimpaired by substances. We would add that a certain degree of anxiety can be beneficial: it will spur you to prepare before your exam and to remain alert during it. We do not advocate the use of any drug, and we suggest consideration of propranolol only for the rare candidate who would be completely incapable of performing without it. It should be taken only under the supervision of a competent physician (other than the candidate!) and only by individuals who have no health problems that would contraindicate its use.

A Day at the Boards

With 500 or more candidates showing up, Part II of the ABPN may at first seem like pandemonium. In actuality, the mechanics of this exam are carefully planned and well coordinated, but that fact may not prevent you from feeling confused and anxious. You can limit the amount of confusion and anxiety you feel, but you'll have to be well organized yourself to do it.

Registration

Registration will usually be held the day before the actual exam. You'll want to be on time. But, just as in the Army, you'll probably hurry up and wait—wait to get your forms, wait for information, and wait for your hotel room. In fact, while you are waiting in line for your room key, you may find yourself standing shoulder to shoulder with friends and colleagues who are there not to take the exam but to administer it. Fraternizing with examiners can cause discomfort all around, so it's usually better not to try to engage them much in conversation.

You will be given a packet of instructions when you register. You should read it thoroughly (you'll have plenty of opportunity while you're waiting in one of those lines) to check for last-minute changes, bus schedules, and the like. This is when you will learn the exact times of each exam and whether you will have the live patient exam first or second. You will also learn who the team leader of your examiners will be. Other candidates may tell you that some team leaders are reputed to eat candidates for breakfast. Remember that fanciful rumors are usually rife in high-anxiety situations. Although it is true that at one time some directors had reputations for being difficult and demanding, the ABPN now has many checks and balances on attitude and performance. Your best course is to disregard all rumors and believe only what you read and what Board officials tell you.

You and your fellow candidates will be divided into groups for an orientation lecture. You should listen to it carefully, even if it seems only to repeat what you have previously read. Anxiety or confusion could cause you to have trouble absorbing what you read; a second sensory input may help you retain vital information.

The Big Day

Before leaving your room, be sure that you have the packet of information (including map and time schedule) you were given the day before, a pocket package of tissues, propranolol (assuming that you've had experience with it before), and a good book (not psychiatry) that will hold your attention while you wait. Unless you've arranged for late checkout, you might leave your bag with the concierge, where you can retrieve it after the exams. (Although you could take your belongings with you to the exam site, there is usually no safe place provided for storage. You could carry the bag into the exam room with you, but you might feel awkward with it.)

Your information packet should make it clear which bus to take to your first exam. If by mistake you arrive at the wrong examination site, there might not be enough time to find the right one, and you could forfeit the exam. If you aren't absolutely certain, ask the driver before you board. Most buses make several stops, so double-check to be sure you get off at the right place.

Here's another word of caution about the buses. Candidates sometimes become terribly worried that they won't find the right bus, that it will break down or be hijacked, or that other improbable mishaps will occur. Some then consider driving themselves to the exam site. If you feel tempted to drive, banish the thought at once. The bus has a much better chance of getting you there intact and on time than you do yourself, especially if you are driving in a strange city. Among the saddest Board examination stories we've heard are those of candidates who decided to provide their own transportation, then got lost or couldn't find a parking spot, and thus forfeited their exams.

When you arrive, go at once to your first examination station. This could be either the videotape session or the patient interview. Follow the signs and arrows to the area where you will be examined. This area will probably be identified with the name of the team leader to whom you have been assigned, so follow the arrows to, for example, "Freud's team." The two dozen or more examiners who constitute Freud's team may already be at work, but there will be signs indicating where you are to wait. While you are doing so, check your assignment sheet to be absolutely sure that you are in the right location. We have seen candidates arrive early and wait placidly, only to be told at the last moment that they have been waiting for the wrong exam.

After the first exam, get to the next exam site right away. If this means that you must travel to a different facility, take the next available bus. You may feel less anxious once you have made the trek and have located the rooms you will be using.

You might as well relax: you might have to wait as long as several hours between exams. Have lunch, if it's that time, taking care to avoid excessive caffeine or liquids. (One candidate forgot this, and drank so much coffee for lunch that he felt "wired" throughout the afternoon session.) If you have hours to kill, you'll probably feel better if you move around a bit. Consider taking a walk, even if it's only down to the hospital canteen. For distraction, try dipping into the novel you brought along.

You may feel some degree of letdown between exams; some candidates report feelings of actual dissociation. This letdown may be heightened if you must wait for your second examination. (Although the Board tries to schedule things as conveniently as possible for you, with over 500 candidates to accommodate, some will inevitably have schedules that are less than ideal.) If you can find a quiet spot, you might try relaxation exercises or meditation, if that sort of thing has helped you in the past. Even something as simple as taking off your shoes for awhile may refresh you.

Some candidates have reported how difficult they find it to clear their minds of the first exam in time for the second. Those who have this trouble complain that ruminating about mistakes they might have made earlier prevents them from concentrating fully on the second exam. If you are worried about this happening to you, you might spend some of your time between exams writing down your recollections, anxieties, and questions on a piece of paper. Sealing that paper in an envelope and mailing it to yourself may help you achieve the desired distance from the first exam.

You may see candidates poring over psychiatric texts. Don't let that get you down: there's nothing anyone will learn from a textbook in the next hour or two that will help significantly during an oral exam.

Conversation with a fellow candidate could pass the time, provided you can find one who isn't too nervous and doesn't talk shop. It will probably be of little use to talk with other candidates about the previous exam. You won't learn much that will help you with your own exam, and any "information" you gather may be so distorted by anxiety and misperception as to be worse than worthless. Some candidates have been trapped by what they were told a videotape would contain, only to discover that the tape had been changed for the later exams.

Chapter 4 ─────────────────────────

The Examiners

Selecting the Examiners

During your 2 examination hours you will have direct contact with at least six and probably seven or eight examiners. That may seem to be a lot, but it's under 3% of those who will be working that session. Who are all these psychiatrists, and how are they chosen to participate in this exercise that is so vitally important to you?

There is only one absolute qualification for prospective ABPN examiners: each has earned the same certificate in psychiatry that you are being examined for. That certificate, plus a curriculum vitae and a letter from the interested individual to the Board, will win the aspiring examiner a spot on the computerized list of potential participants. In that sense, the process has a considerable element of self-selection.

The way the panel is made up risks underrepresenting certain groups such as private practitioners, who may feel they cannot afford the time to conduct examinations. Female psychiatrists are also more likely to decline an invitation to examine at any given session, though according to Dr. Stephen Scheiber, the Board's executive secretary, this tendency may have eased in the past few years. But the Board strives for fair representation; some first-time examiners were candidates themselves only a year or two before. They remember well how it feels to be in your shoes.

Choosing a Team

To help you understand how the exams are run, we'll look at how the examination teams are structured for each of the smaller exams given every year. (Details of the history and makeup of the ABPN are given in Appendix A.) (Each of these exams involves about 400 psychiatrist candidates. The larger exam, given once yearly, involves about twice the number of examiners and candidates.)

The selection process begins with the eight directors of the ABPN who are psychiatrists. Each director leads a team. When more teams are needed, as is the case for the larger exam (when up to 20 might be required), former directors of the Board are asked to participate.

Each team leader will choose four senior, or "floating," examiners. These highly experienced examiners form the stable nucleus of each director's examiner team. Many of the team members travel to two or even all three of the exam sessions each year. With four senior examiners needed for each of eight teams, each of the smaller examinations will require a minimum of 32 senior examiners.

Thus, each team is made up of a director (team leader), senior examiners (also known as floaters), and primary examiners.

The primary examiners spend the most time with the candidates; it is principally on their opinions that the fate of each candidate ultimately rests. How are these primary examiners chosen?

To keep travel costs and inconvenience to a minimum, primary examiners are selected from geographic areas as near as possible to the exam site. From the computerized list (1,200 names as of this writing) of psychiatrists who previously were examiners or who have been recommended to the Board as potential examiners, each director chooses about 40 primary examiners, ranking them in order of preference. A computer program then selects the top 25 or so from each director's list. These physicians will be invited to be examiners during that particular session.

Now, we have described all of those who will participate in your examination. For one of the two smaller exams, each of 8 directors works closely with 4 senior examiners (32 total). Each senior examiner oversees 4 primary examiners (128 in all), who work in pairs with the candidates. Therefore, this smaller session requires 168 certified psychiatrists to examine just over twice that number of candidates.

Examiners are not paid for their time. They are reimbursed for transportation expenses and are given a per diem allowance for hotel and meals. Except for their lost income, they just about break even for the event. Whether they seem warm or aloof, whether they are relaxed or intense in their questioning, all of them remember the months of diligent preparation and anxiety that preceded their own Board examinations. As Maleson et al. (1980) noted, most examiners "struggle for clarity and fairness in their questions and privately empathize with the candidates."

Examiners and the Exam

To ensure that you are judged fairly, each hour of your examination will be witnessed in its entirety by two examiners—the primary examiners—and in part by the senior examiner, who moves back and forth between two candidates. Team leaders (directors) will also drop in to sign your attendance card and to observe each candidate firsthand; some may spend considerable time with a few candidates so as to evaluate the performance of examiners. At the end of the entire testing session, directors will use the grade cards and their own observations to help judge the effectiveness of individual primary examiners. This information will be used to assist the Board in choosing examination teams for subsequent years.

A rookie examiner will usually be paired with one who is more experienced. On most teams, examiners will also change partners after each morning and afternoon session. Over the course of 2 days, each examining psychiatrist will thus be able to observe the examining styles of four colleagues. Within each pair of primary examiners, one will often take the responsibility for asking most of the questions. Partners generally will alternate this responsibility with each successive candidate.

In preparing for each testing session, examiners scan the candidates for familiar names or faces. Should your prospective examiner know you, you will be shifted to another pair of primary examiners. You should also tell the team leader if you know either of the examiners to whom you have been assigned. This way, no examiner will be placed in the untenable position of having to pass judgment on a friend or acquaintance, and you will feel that you have received as unbiased an exam as possible.

Other than your name, the primary examiners know little about you. If they see your attendance card, they may know where you live, but that's all. Specifically, they know nothing of your practice (private, institutional, academic), your theoretical orientation (if any), or your training. They have not been told whether this is your first time at the exams, or whether you are repeating Part II. There is intent in all this ignorance: it is to avoid any appearance of prejudice that might result if the examiner had personal information about you. As a matter of fact, examiners are forbidden to ask *any* personal or professional questions that are not related to the exam. This is one reason some may seem cool or uninterested in you.

How Grading Works

After you leave the room, your examiners have four tasks:

1. For every category on your grade card (we'll list them all later in this chapter) they circle a *preliminary grade.* For the first two categories of the patient

interview (Physician-Patient Relationship and Conduct of the Interview), this grade can be only a pass or fail. For the remaining categories of the patient interview and for all categories of the videotape examination, the grade can be Pass, High Condition, Low Condition, or Fail. Of course, such a system means that the first two categories are weighted more heavily than the others.

2. For each of these categories, the examiners make notes that document your performance.

3. Without consulting one another, the two examiners independently record their individual impressions of your *overall performance* in the form of a grade: Pass, Condition, or Fail. (The terms *High Condition* and *Low Condition* are not used to describe overall performance or for the consensus grade, which we describe next.)

4. Finally, the primary examiners compare notes to reach a *consensus grade* of Pass, Condition, or Fail. In most cases, they agree at once; however, if they do not see eye to eye, they do their best to arrive at a consensus grade through discussion. If they cannot agree, the senior examiner, who has been in and out of the room during the examination, acts as a mediator and attempts to reconcile the vote.

Otherwise, senior examiners are usually willing to defer to the judgment of the primary examiners. Maleson et al. (1980) noted that "In . . . marginal cases the several examiners who have observed the candidate typically spend extra time and energy in vigorous and sometimes agonized debate."

If ever these three examiners cannot arrive at a consensus grade, the team leader might get involved. This seldom happens. In fact, Maleson et al. noted that examiners' assessments are surprisingly similar, even before any discussion takes place.

Finally, once the decisions on both the videotape and the live patient exam have been made, they are put together for the *final grade*. Here is how that is done:

Throughout the day, entire teams work together in pairs. While Director A's team is testing candidates 1 through 48 on the videotape, Director B's team will be testing this same group of candidates on the live patient examination. (On the second day, team A will do the patient exam and team B will do the videotape exam. This helps keep examiners fresh.) In the evening, director A and director B compare notes on the day's 48 candidates to arrive at a consensus final score. Now there can be only Pass or Fail; Condition is not an option as a final grade.

If both grades are a Pass, the candidate passes the exam. If either of the two grades is Fail or if both grades are a Condition, the candidate fails and must retake all of Part II. If one grade is a Pass and the other a Condition, the comments on the grade cards are scrutinized. If these comments indicate that on one exam the candidate passed with flying colors and on the other had a Condition that was not too low, the two directors will check to see that the areas of weakness that occasioned the Condition were handled satisfactorily on the other exam. If that was the case, they will usually raise the Condition grade to a Pass. This helps explain why a Condition is more likely to be raised to a Pass on the videotape portion than on the live patient examination: a poor interview cannot be redeemed on the videotape exam.

If the Condition is raised to Pass and the other grade was already Pass, then the overall Part II grade will also be a Pass. However, should the grade card notes indicate that the Condition was really close to a Failure or that the Pass bordered on a Condition, the candidate may be judged too marginal. Then, usually after much discussion and anguish, the final grade for the entire exam will be a Failure.

How Do Examiners Prepare?

If you read Appendix A, you will see from the candidate's perspective how the exams have changed through the years. But Part II of the Boards has been undergoing constant evolution for the examiners, as well.

The most notable change in recent years has been a concerted effort to give first-time examiners formal training in the philosophy and methods of examination technique. Since 1979, first timers (and old hands who have not examined for 2 years or more) are asked to report half a day early for a special training session. During this orientation session, held on the morning of the day before the first exam, examiners are given a description of the criteria for the various performance areas. Each criterion is explored and defined in detail by the examination teams. Team members are not usually close colleagues, so this review of rules and general group discussion tends to moderate extreme positions and develop consensus as to the level of performance expected of a Board diplomat. New examiners also have the opportunity to participate as both examiner and candidate in a mock board examination. (Many new examiners have remarked how anxiety provoking even this benign exercise can be.)

That afternoon all examiners, regardless of experience, gather to view the videotapes that will be used during the following 2 days. After the viewing, the entire group discusses these tapes to develop consensus as to psychopathology, differential diagnosis, most likely diagnosis, possible treatment plans, and other important data that should be apparent from the tapes. Rules of scoring, changes in the exam procedure, and other pertinent matters are reviewed. In all, new examiners spend 8 hours and experienced examiners spend 3 hours preparing for the work of the following 2 days.

Written Instructions to Examiners

All examiners are given a set of detailed, written instructions to help ensure a fair and uniform approach to the candidates. In this section, we paraphrase the latest version of these instructions (the wording, though not the spirit, changes from year to year) so that you can better understand what your examiners expect of you. Much of this material will be familiar to you, but we'll repeat some of it so that you will have the clearest picture possible of what your examiners will be told. (We have occasionally added an editorial comment to underline information that seems especially important.)

The written instructions begin with a reminder that you will be examined for a total of 2 hours, 1 hour each with an actual patient and with a videotape. Because you have already passed Part I of the exam, which covers clinical neurology and basic science as it relates to neurology and psychiatry, you will only be examined in the clinical aspects of psychiatry.

The examiners will emphasize problems that are clinically relevant and practical. They will avoid trivia such as, "Who was the only psychiatrist ever awarded a Nobel prize in medicine?"[1] Part II of the Boards should focus principally on the clinical data and problems detailed in the interview. Most of the questions should stem from your experience with your patient; any supplementary questions should be clinical. Your examiners are reminded to give you enough time to discuss different management plans. They are not to expect a specific diagnosis—rather, a working impression with its attendant differential diagnosis.

The standard that will be used for judging you is clearly set out: the only criterion is that of general clinical competence in the care of psychiatric patients. This term is explicitly defined as the abilities to

- Gather information
- Use the information to arrive at a coherent diagnosis
- Decide about treatment and management of the patient
- Recognize, understand, and manage clinical problems

You must show that you can do the following:

- Elicit and interpret signs and symptoms
- Apply clinical skills to clinical problems
- Make appropriate diagnoses

---

1 Julius Wagner von Jauregg, in 1927, for fever treatment of general paresis of the insane.

- Apply proper therapy
- Set priorities
- Recognize and deal with problems resulting from therapy

In judging your overall performance, examiners are asked to evaluate whether they would accept you as a colleague. They are reminded that once you have been certified as a specialist by the ABPN, you are presented to the public as a qualified psychiatrist.

Examiners are specifically warned about possible criteria that could—but will not—be used in judging you. These include the demonstration of unusual excellence, the possession of academic skills (such as the ability to teach or do research), the ability to perform in your own job, and adherence to any particular theoretical model or school of psychiatry.

General Examination Procedures

Here is what your examiners have been told about the day's activities:

Each session, morning and afternoon, comprises three examinations. This is the schedule:

8:30–9:30
9:50–10:50
11:10–12:10
LUNCH
1:10–2:10
2:30–3:30
3:50–4:50

Examiners are cautioned neither to release you early nor to keep you past the end of an examination hour, but to adhere exactly to the schedule. Bus schedules and other examinations depend on it.

Examiners are not to evaluate you if they already know you. If they even suspect prior acquaintance, they are to disqualify themselves from working with you.

You will be attended by two primary examiners for the entire hour; senior examiners and team leaders will occasionally enter or leave the room. Examiners are reminded to share the interview time with one another. Sometime during the second examination, the ABPN director who is the team leader of your section will collect the registration card bearing your picture that you have been carrying.

A feature of the examination that is particularly emphasized with the examiners is stress. Examiners are reminded how anxiety provoking an oral examination can be, and they are requested to do all they can to minimize the effects of anxiety on you. As the examiner orientation instructions state: "It is the examiner's job to help the candidate to display competence in what might be best described as an environment of compassionate collegial neutrality."

At the beginning of the half-hour question-and-answer period, most examiners will offer you a minute or two to collect your thoughts. If your examiners forget to do this and you feel you need the time, you may ask for it.

Examiners are reminded that it is better to begin with a relatively specific question (such as "Please summarize this patient"). More open-ended questions (such as "What did you think of the patient?") contain too little structure and have been known to make candidates feel overwhelmed with anxiety. It is appropriate to ask candidates to "present the patient and mental status examination, then give a formulation of the history, finally moving on to a differential diagnosis and recommendations for further workup and management." (In any event, it is good advice to summarize the information from the interview you conducted or observed, highlighting the demonstrated pathology, and then to present concisely the information from the mental status examination.)

Examiners' attitudes toward you should be characterized by professionalism, respect, and cordiality. They are specifically reminded not to appear sarcastic, hostile, or condescending. They must maintain utmost confidentiality and must refrain from discussing you or the examination in public places—no gossiping in hallways, hotel lobbies, rest rooms, or buses. They must not eat, drink, or smoke while they are with you, and they must neither signal one another nor attempt to interview the patient themselves.

Examiners are to maintain this demeanor while revealing nothing to you about your performance. Specifically, examiners must not ask you any personal questions and must avoid any conversation that might seem prejudicial. (Obviously, this requirement involves trying to keep an almost impossibly delicate balance.) Examiners are to be friendly but neutral in their responses. They must avoid statements or behavior that might seem to comment on how you are doing: an inopportune smile or statement such as "That's fine" might give you a false sense of security. At the same time, examiners are asked to avoid being cold or unresponsive because that, too, could signal something that is not intended and may heighten your anxiety.

Your examiners are reminded not to teach, and they will not give you feedback. Should you ask them to say how you are doing or to tell you the correct answer, they are supposed to respond that the rules prohibit answers to such questions. (Anyway, the examiners are not looking for a right answer, but rather for your discussion of the issues raised by the patient or videotape.) Your examiners should avoid long silences; if you seem to be perplexed, they should rephrase a question to help you out.

Examiners are supposed to focus on finding out what you know, rather than what you do not know. They are asked to cover several different areas in the course of the half hour. Once they have found that you do not know something, they should move on to another area, rather than belaboring an issue that has already been determined. They are also asked not to limit their questions to areas of their own special interest, but to be broad based in their investigation of your abilities. They are specifically requested not to ask progressively more difficult questions in one area until you reach a point where you can no longer answer. This tactic only increases anxiety and serves no useful testing purpose.

The examiners are to use the full 60 minutes, at the end of which your examination will be completed. If this was your first exam, you will be sent on to the next one. If it was your second (and final) exam, you may then leave.

The Live Patient Session

The examiners are asked to give especially close attention to the patient interview, because it is the only point in the entire certification process at which they can evaluate your interviewing and interpersonal skills. The ABPN prescribes a number of procedural rules for examiners to follow:

When you enter the room with the examiners, the patient should already be there waiting. You should be allowed to arrange seating in the room as you wish.

The patients should have already been told that the purpose of this examination is to test you, the candidate. They will have signed an informed consent form to this effect. Inpatients may be rewarded with additional ward privileges or a small amount of money. Outpatients may receive money to cover their travel expenses.

The examiners should remind you that you will have 30 minutes to interview your patient. They should tell you that they will signal when you have only 5 minutes left.

Charts are not supplied. You and the examiners start with the same information about the patient, which is usually none at all. (Occasionally, a patient will be interviewed by more than one candidate; then, a pair of examiners may have information from a previous interview. They are not to let this information influence their evaluation of your performance.)

You may take notes (but see our advice on this subject in Chapters 5 and 11). You will not be allowed to do a physical examination. If you think that one is necessary, you can discuss this point after the patient has left the room.

Examiners are asked not to intervene during your interview unless some clear emergency arises. Examiners will not terminate the patient interview early. If you try to end the interview before the full half hour has elapsed, they should advise you against it.

But what if the patient should attempt to leave before the interview is over?

How you handle this situation (see Chapter 5) will be assessed by the examiners as a part of their evaluation of you. Should you be unable to persuade the patient to stay, and it is still early in the session, they will try to obtain another patient for you. If it is too late in the session for another patient, or if none is available, you will be asked to review what happened and to discuss what might have motivated the patient to leave.

After the patient interview has been completed, one of the examiners will see to it that the patient is safely returned to the care of the clinical staff at the facility.

The Videotape Examination

Examiners are reminded that the film is a stimulus and is not intended as a paragon of interviewing technique. They are advised that discussing the interview's quality, even though it might be relevant, can be a distraction. It is acknowledged that the videotape data are often ambiguous and that such a discussion could prove more distracting than relevant. Based on the taped interview, it is fair to ask all manner of questions, including those that relate to your own skills of observation and judgment. Any supplementary questions should be clinically oriented.

The focus of the videotape exam is your observations, differential diagnosis, treatment plans, and prognosis. The examiners will judge the appropriateness of your plan for managing the patient. They may also ask what information you would look for if you were interviewing the videotaped patient. They are reminded that the lack of opportunity to observe your interaction with the patient may make it harder to evaluate the videotape examination than the one that follows the live patient interview.

The examiners will give you adequate time to discuss various plans of management. You will not be expected to make a specific final diagnosis, but instead to choose a working impression with an associated differential diagnosis.

Grading Time

Grading of Part II is the responsibility of primary and senior examiners as well as of the directors. It occurs in four stages:

- Subcategory grade (given by individual examiners)
- Preliminary grade (also given by individual examiners)
- Consensus grade (combined judgment of the two primary examiners)
- Final grade for the entire examination

Here is what your examiners will be told about the grading system:

First, all primary examiners record subcategory grades and support them with written documentation that may include direct quotes from your responses during the examination itself. The subcategories for the patient examination are

- Physician-patient relationship
- Conduct of interview
- Organization and presentation of data
- Phenomenology, diagnosis, and prognosis
- Etiologic, pathogenic, and therapeutic issues (divided into biological, psychological, and social categories)

The subcategories for the videotape examination are quite similar. They are

- Observation of data
- Organization and presentation of data
- Phenomenology, diagnosis, and prognosis
- Etiologic, pathogenic, and therapeutic issues (divided into categories similar to those for the patient exam)

The Grades

The basic grades for the entire grading process are Pass, Condition, and Fail. Before every exam, directors will present the following definitions to all examiners in their sections. The directors and their senior examiners will do all they can to ensure grades that are consistent. They will not give instructions that would bend the rules beyond a strict application of the definitions. This means that no one will suggest to examiners that they should try to pass, condition, or fail a certain percentage of candidates.

A grade of Pass means that for that subcategory or examination you have met at least the minimal standards expected of a competent psychiatric specialist.

Condition is a borderline grade that ultimately will be either raised or lowered, depending on what other grades you receive. It is used when the examiners don't think they have enough information to warrant a Pass or when they worry that you might have some specific deficiency. The grades High Condition and Low Condition are used only by the individual primary examiners in rating the subcategory performances; later, they will use these grades to support the overall preliminary grade. High Condition means that the performance is borderline, but close to a Pass; Low Condition means that the performance is close to an outright Failure.

A consensus grade of Fail on either the patient or the videotape examination will always result in an overall failure, and you would have to take Part II again to be certified.

The Grading Process

For most subcategories of either the patient or the videotape examination, primary examiners may list any of four grades: Pass, High Condition, Low Condition, or Fail. On the live patient exam, a Condition cannot be given for subcategories involving the interview itself (conduct of the interview and the physician-patient relationship); only Pass or Fail can be used.

After the subcategory grades have been recorded by the individual primary examiners, each of them records a preliminary grade of Pass, Condition, or Fail. Examiners are told that the preliminary grades they award should reflect the subcategory grades, but that they don't have to be mathematically exact. Here are some examples: a candidate who is given subcategory grades of two High Conditions and three Low Conditions would be given a preliminary grade of Condition. A candidate who receives subcategory grades of two Passes and three High Conditions could be given a preliminary grade of either Pass or Condition. The choice would depend on the judgment of the individual examiner.

Next, the two primary examiners confer to arrive at a consensus (again, Pass, Condition, or Fail). Although their grades for the subcategories need not be identical, the two primary examiners must agree on a final grade. They are reminded that your performance must be carefully documented in writing, because these grade cards are used by the directors to determine the final grade for the entire Part II examination and for later review should you appeal a grade of Fail. If the two primary examiners, even with the help of the senior examiner, cannot agree on a Pass or Fail, they may give you a Condition for that part of the exam. This practice is implicitly discouraged by pointing out that the directors and senior examiners, who must decide how to count a Condition in the final grading process, know the candidate less well than do the two primary examiners.

Examiners are encouraged to write down as much data as possible; terse generalizations have no value for the later grading sessions. These written descriptions should include *verbatim* responses and concrete examples of your strengths as well as your weaknesses. Prejudicial comments of a personal, racial, ethnic, or sexist nature are explicitly prohibited. Whatever consensus grade they may give, primary examiners are asked to discuss the grade with the senior examiner and to mention your specific weaknesses and strengths. Any instances of unprofessional or unethical conduct (admittedly rare) are to be brought immediately to the attention of the director and to be documented carefully on the grade cards.

At a later grading session, the consensus grades from the videotape and patient examinations are inspected by the directors of the ABPN, and a final grade of either Pass or Fail (no Conditions here) is determined. At the final grading conference, the directors bring together the results of the consensus grades on the videotape and patient exams. If you receive a grade of Condition on one exam but pass the other, the directors can (and usually will) raise your final grade to a Pass.

The following grade combinations will result in a Fail for the entire Part II examination:

Pass-Fail
Condition-Condition
Condition-Fail
Fail-Fail
Pass-Condition (unless the Pass is strong enough to raise the Condition
   to a Pass)

The final grade must be ratified by vote of the entire Board.

Finally, examiners are reminded to keep each candidate's performance in strict confidence. They are not to tell you how you have done, either during or after the exam. If they are contacted by a candidate, they are to refer all questions to the ABPN office in Deerfield, Illinois.

Chapter 5 ——————————————————————

Exam Etiquette

Interviewing a patient for the psychiatry Boards may be one of the most difficult challenges you'll have to face as a fully trained physician. The reason is
simple. Compared with every other clinical interview, you are entering a world
turned upside-down. Normally, you are the examiner; today, you are the examined. And, in a sense, the patient is a part of the examining team—and knows it.
This can be very disconcerting! But most trials seem worse in prospect than in
aspect, and in that sense this one is no different. Once you get going and sink
into your comfortable interview routine, you'll probably find that the real thing
is little worse than the mock boards you have already experienced.

The Patient's Comfort

Candidates occasionally feel sorry for what their patients must put up with. But
the patient's state of mind is usually pretty placid compared with that of many
candidates. Board exam patients are all volunteers. Most are offered a small sum
of money—perhaps $10—to compensate for child care or for travel expenses to
the examination site. (To avoid the appearance of unfairness, inpatients also are
usually offered a small sum. But if the treating physician feels this would work
against the treatment program, the pay might instead be contributed to the patients' general fund.)

Even without pay, most patients report that helping psychiatrists qualify for
certification is at least interesting and sometimes beneficial. In a study by Rosen
et al. (1979), nearly all patients felt they had been treated with courtesy and respect. Although some of these hospitalized patients found the experience stressful, careful preparation by staff members probably helped the majority to view

their participation in positive terms. Rosen and colleagues thought that the examination increased patients' self-esteem by giving them an opportunity to use their psychiatric difficulties in an adaptive manner.

The patients described by Eveloff and McCreary (1972) also said that they were glad they could make a contribution. "Even though I found [the interviews] mildly unpleasant, I think I benefited from the experience," one patient commented. "I found it fun," said another. Still another patient remarked, "I wouldn't mind being in another one. . . . I believe that talking to different people about my problems usually helps me. . . ." Altogether, Board examination patients deserve our gratitude; pity would be misplaced.

Both of the studies cited above mention that patients are often astute in their assessments of the different candidates and may bring considerable compassion of their own to the interview situation: "The poor [doctors] seemed so nervous that I was wondering in what way I could help them." Thus, many patients come to the examination with built-in support for you, the candidate. Your job may be less to provide for your patient's comfort than to show your examiners that you know how to put patients at their ease and that their comfort is important to you.

At the beginning of your examination, when your anxiety level is at its highest, putting the patient at ease may seem like a tall order. But you can use the normal routine of these first few moments to reduce your anticipatory anxiety. Just before you begin, rather than thinking about the length of the hour that stretches before you, focus instead on the physical routine of the introduction. Even if you wonder whether anxiety will prevent you from concentrating well enough to take a decent history, you'll gain confidence from your ability to make introductions, shake hands all around, and make sure the patient is comfortably seated. (Because there will be considerable traffic in and out of the room, your primary examiners will probably see to it that the chair nearest the door is left vacant.) Anxiety could reduce your repertoire of responses, but responding normally in a familiar situation can reduce your anxiety.

Getting Started

Introduce yourself and learn the patient's name. You may introduce the patient to the examiners, or you may decide to ignore this nicety. Some examiners introduce themselves, but all wear name tags, so you can't go wrong. Either way, you won't be faulted if at least you point out their function to the patient.

You might start off by saying that you appreciate the patient's help with the exam. That you are being examined should have been explained before, but the patient may have forgotten. A simple "Thank you" will also help enlist sympathy and cooperation for the half hour ahead.

All of these preliminaries will take perhaps half a minute. In those 30 seconds, you should also observe the patient's general appearance, gait, facial expressions, and handshake. As you begin your clinical observations, your own anxiety should diminish further.

You may feel fenced in. The room you will occupy for the next hour could be less than ideal for a patient interview. Try to put it out of your mind. You don't want to waste precious time commenting on the ambience of some place you must endure for an hour and then never see again.

Although its appointments may be spartan, at a minimum the room will be furnished with a desk (or table) and several chairs. If you can, try to arrange your own chair so that only a corner of the desk is between you and the patient. This allows you maximum flexibility to change the distance between you and the patient, as the content of the interview dictates.

Interacting With the Patient

Your interactions with the patient during the next half hour will be determined by several factors. Besides your physical proximity, already mentioned, the diagnostic and personality characteristics of the patient and the content of the interview will play important roles. Of these, the patient's demeanor is most likely to shape the interview.

Your Patient's Affect

If the patient is depressed or anxious, you will probably respond automatically with warmth and comforting words. A manic patient may cause you to become more cheerful and ebullient yourself. On the other hand, hostility or suspiciousness may cause you to lean further back in your chair. You may even want to move it a few inches away to help the patient maintain a distance that is more comfortable for both of you.

It is appropriate (and expected) that you show signs of sympathy. You will do this largely through facial expressions—you don't have time for more than the briefest of verbal blandishments. As in any other clinical situation, be careful not to censure the patient. Refrain from frowning, grimacing, or showing other signs of disapproval should your patient discuss sexual behavior, substance abuse, or other matters you don't approve of.

Your examiners will note how you respond to signs of distress. As in any clinical interview, patients sometimes cry. You can deal silently with tearfulness by offering your pocket pack of facial tissues. This is a speedy, appropriate fix that won't disrupt the flow of information. But tailor your interview accordingly; when the patient is crying is no time to ask for serial 7s.

Anxiety may prompt other requests from the patient that you can't satisfy so easily—to smoke a cigarette while being interviewed, for example. Most medical facilities today won't allow smoking indoors anyway, and you can fall back on the absence of an ashtray or the presence of prohibitory signs as reasons for refusing. If smoking is prohibited, you may be able to put the patient off with the promise of "just a few more minutes, then you can go." If not, take a deep breath and plunge ahead, telling yourself that, just this once, failing to get information would be more harmful than secondhand smoke.

Patients may feel stressed if they think they are performing poorly, so watch out for restlessness or other signs of anxiety should your patient have trouble recalling historical information or completing portions of the mental status examination. You can acknowledge the stress and offer some simple reassurance. Try: "You're telling me exactly what I want to know" or "Nearly everyone has some problems with subtracting 7s." Should the task prove too frustrating, you could offer a substitute, such as counting backward from 20. Remember that praise can be helpful if it is deserved, but that no one likes to be patronized. Offer reassurance if it is heartfelt and based on reality, but not as a substitute for real understanding.

You will build a working relationship more rapidly if you keep eye contact with your patient. Eye contact will be better if you avoid looking up when the director or senior examiner enters or leaves the room. If you keep your gaze where it ought to be—on the patient—it will help focus the patient's concentration, too.

Should You Take Notes?

Eye contact may be better if you don't take notes. In the context of an examination, note taking can be a time waster. (How much time do you suppose you'll have to review them?) Most examiners accept the fact that a few notes can aid an anxious candidate's memory in a stressful situation. But more than a few notes can interfere with the process of the interview. Your patient may notice that you are writing, and slow down to accommodate your pace. That is one way you could obtain less information. Another is that you will witness less of your patient's own expressions and body language—which the examiners will be noting carefully.

At most, make one-word notes to remind you of topics to pursue later on.

And use a single sheet of paper: some candidates bury themselves in a snow-storm of memo-sized note papers that seem to distract more than they could ever help.

Once you have finished discussing the case with your examiners, they will collect any notes you have made. This provides two sorts of protection: it ensures the confidentiality of the patient and reduces your ability to reconstruct the interview later, should you dispute the results of your Board examination. The confiscated notes will be discarded; examiners do not use them to help determine your grade.

Talk the Same Language

As with any other interview, you will get more information if you tailor your conversational style to the age and background of the patient. Slang expressions that are "cool" or "rad" might invite the confidence of a teenager, but might create an unnecessary gulf between you and an older patient. If the patient's educational level is considerably less than yours or if you and the patient come from different ethnic backgrounds, you should be especially careful to speak clearly and simply. You could be the greatest interviewer since Emil Kraepelin, but if this particular patient doesn't understand you, you might as well be speaking German.

Also in the interest of clarity, be sure to avoid psychiatric jargon. Most patients haven't taken psychology courses, so they may not understand even simple terms such as *psychosis* and *mania*. When you inquire about concepts such as these, don't leave it to the patient to decide what you mean. Instead, describe the behavior or concept in simple English. To do otherwise invites three unpleasant results: 1) you'll get less information, 2) you won't build rapport, and 3) your examiners will fault you for poor communication.

You must also work hard to understand what the patient means. Although a social drink to you may be a glass of Perrier with a twist, to your patient it may mean a six-pack of beer after work. What does the patient mean by "black beauties?" How much heroin is there in a "nickel bag?" If the patient uses psychiatric jargon, does it mean the same thing to both of you? For example, in the street vernacular *paranoid* may simply mean fearful, with no connotation of psychosis.

If you and your patient have different accents, it could add to the burden of understanding one another. You should probably be candid about this problem. Acknowledge right at the outset that you come from different parts of the country (or world) and that you both may have to work a little harder to communicate. Don't imply that it is the patient who is hard to understand—that would put you on opposite sides of the issue. The spirit you want to convey is that you are working together to achieve a common goal. And don't hesitate to ask for repetition if you need it. If you didn't understand the patient, the examiners probably didn't either, and everyone will benefit from the clarification.

Personal Matters

In some parts of the country, therapists commonly refer to patients by first names. Regardless of what you do in the privacy of your own office, for the purposes of the Board examination address your patient by title and last name: Mr., Mrs., Miss, or Ms. Smith. Even if you are old enough to be the patient's parent, doing otherwise (especially on first acquaintance) suggests condescension. The title and last name approach is professional, and it encourages the patient to refer to you as "Doctor." This will help you maintain a respectful distance from the patient, something in which the examiners will be interested. Here is one possible exception to the last-name rule: if your patient insists that you use a first name or nickname, don't waste time arguing. Acquiesce, and explain later during the discussion.

As a general rule, we believe that it is permissible for psychiatrists and other therapists to reveal something of themselves to their patients once they have become well acquainted. In the everyday practice of psychiatry, a bit of human interaction has little to lose and much to gain in terms of rapport, confidence, and compliance. But in the context of your Board examination, sharing personal information is usually just plain wrong. For one thing, you haven't time for anything other than business. For another, your examiner's ideas of what personal information you could reveal to a patient may be quite different from your own. Finally, you probably won't have much permanent effect—positive or negative—on your Board examination patient, whom you are unlikely to see ever again. Stick to the business at hand, which is to pass this exam. If you are feeling anxious, don't talk about it (unless the patient comments on your jitters, in which case you are probably better off with a graceful acknowledgment). If you share a birthday or a taste in clothing with your patient, keep it to yourself.

You should also keep your own negative emotions private. For example, don't let anxiety cause you to talk too much; any time you spend talking is time the patient cannot be giving you information. And no matter what the provocation, be sure not to lose your temper. We agree that that is pretty unlikely to happen. But a particularly obnoxious, recalcitrant, vague, or otherwise difficult patient would raise anybody's hackles. If you are given such a patient, you may need to exercise considerable restraint to keep your reactions professional.

What about the positive emotions? Although smiling is just fine (even recommended for putting a patient at ease), don't tell jokes, make puns or ripostes, or regale the patient and examiners with anecdotes. Patients (or examiners) who don't share your sense of humor may think you are having a joke at their expense. But it is quite permissible to respond normally to funny situations. Although we've changed the names, at one exam the dialogue went something like this:

CANDIDATE.   I'd like to introduce the examiners, Dr. Wright and Dr. Wong.
PATIENT.   *[Feeling quite jolly.]*   Oh, do you want to see if I can tell Wright from Wong?
CANDIDATE.   *[Becoming flustered.]*   Well, no, uh, I'm Dr. Hugh.
PATIENT.   Who?
CANDIDATE.   No, Hugh!

By this time, the examiners were beside themselves, the patient was in control of the interview, and the candidate, who might have done better to give in and join the merriment, was ready for therapy.

Active Listening

During the Board examination is no time to affect the "blank screen" attitude of the traditional psychotherapy hour. Neither should you repeat every statement the patient makes. Some candidates do, perhaps out of habit or anxiety, and it's a time waster. Instead, while your patient is talking, practice *active listening*. This involves several verbal and nonverbal techniques.

During the entire interview, you should avoid looking at the examiners. This will help you keep your attention focused solely on the patient and the patient's attention focused solely on you. Let the patient know you are interested by maintaining eye contact. A nod or a smile signals that you are paying attention. You can also show your interest and attention by leaning forward a little to hear about a particularly traumatic event or deep-felt emotion, or by gently shaking your head to sympathize with the frustration you hear expressed about some desperate social situation. An occasional brief comment ("Oh, my!" or "You must have felt awful!") to acknowledge a particularly interesting (or devastating) piece of information may also be appropriate. Regardless of which technique you use, try not to interfere with the flow of information, especially during the early part of the interview. Intervene only when you have to clarify an important point.

Avoid saying something that might add to your patient's burden. One patient told her examiner that her husband had forced sex on her, but didn't know whether that would be considered molestation. "It sure sounds like molestation to me!" exclaimed the candidate, thus potentially further raising anxieties the patient was not yet prepared to deal with. The rule: try to conduct an interview that leaves your patient unchanged when you are finished.

Sensitive Subjects

As in most other psychiatric interviews, you should feel free to ask just about any sort of question. Both you and the patient may feel somewhat uncomfortable about delving into highly sensitive material, especially in front of witnesses. But if you maintain your composure, ignore distractions, and treat the sensitive questions as a matter of routine, your patient will probably do the same.

Personal finances, suicidal ideas and behaviors, substance abuse, and sexual functioning are sensitive areas that can be vital to any psychiatric evaluation. Because of the AIDS epidemic, with its implications for psychiatric diagnosis and human suffering, it is now more important than ever to inquire explicitly about homosexual practices, the use of condoms, specific sexual acts, street drugs, and shared needles. Your discomfort when exploring these areas will be nothing compared with what you would feel later had you not obtained the information.

Lying

What should you do if you think your patient is lying? To begin with, most patients are truthful most of the time. (Some of the data underlying this assumption are reviewed in Haas et al. [1987]). During a brief interview such as this one, it is unusual to have reason to suspect otherwise. Therefore, you should assume that your patient is telling the truth unless you are faced with one of these specific situations:

- The history is inconsistent with the known course of a psychiatric disorder. Example: Years of psychosis and repeated hospitalizations notwithstanding, your patient denies ever receiving neuroleptic medications.
- The history is internally inconsistent. Example: Despite claims of being successfully self-employed in business, your patient mentions receiving welfare checks.
- The discussion turns to any behavior usually associated with shame, guilt, or a need to prevent detection. Examples: Alcohol abuse, illicit drug sales, criminal behavior, and sexual problems.
- You suspect your patient has a diagnosis that can be characterized by lying or deception. Examples: Antisocial personality disorder and factitious disorder with predominantly physical signs and symptoms (Munchausen syndrome).

Playing medical detective can be one of the most satisfying challenges to confront a psychiatrist, but during this exam you probably won't have much opportunity to resolve the doubts that would be raised by the above-mentioned situations. You should not risk losing your patient's interest and cooperation with a confrontation over some historical detail that might be immaterial.

You should, however, try to resolve any confusion you have over information that may represent simple misstatement. For example, you would hate to have the examiners wonder why you failed to ask whether the patient really meant that he had buried—not married—his wife in June. Lesser contradictions and inconsistencies are better saved to discuss after the patient has left the room. Then, you will want to correlate and contrast what you heard with what you saw. Your armchair detecting can be done more impressively—and more safely—after the "evidence" has left the room.

Quitting Time

Terminating the patient interview is an aspect of your half hour that you will want to time right down to the last second. Even if you think you have obtained all the necessary information for a thorough discussion of your patient's diagnosis, management, prognosis, and etiology, you could always obtain more. If you stop the interview early, you may appear arrogant. Perhaps worse, it may seem that you don't recognize the importance of the detailed social history, childhood behavioral traits, or Aunt Gertrude's lifelong problem with blackberry wine. In a half-hour interview, there will always be areas of history that you will be unable, for want of time, to cover thoroughly.

On the other hand, you want to complete the interview gracefully. Your examiners will tell you when you have only 5 minutes left. Keep an eye on your watch, and try to finish up with no time to spare. If in the final minutes you think you've covered everything, you can issue an open-ended invitation: "Is there anything we haven't covered that you think would help me to understand you?" This may start the information flowing again. On the other hand, if you are still gathering information when time runs out, the examiners will ask you to stop. Then, with a handshake and a quick "Thank you" for cooperating with you, usher the patient from the room.

Anxiety, psychosis, anger, or some other stressor will occasionally make a patient try to leave the interview before the time is up. Sometimes backup patients are available and you can start over, but you can't rely on it. Your best protection, of course, is to be so sensitive to the emotions induced by the interview that your patient will be able to endure the entire half hour.

In the uncommon event that the patient tries to leave early, point out that you will need only a "few more minutes" and try to change the subject. Then, your best bet is to take a quick look at the patient's feelings. Acknowledge the anxiety, anger, depression, or fear that may be impelling the patient to leave, and ask for some comments about that emotion. Try an empathic statement such as, "This must be making you feel quite uncomfortable." But take pains to avoid direct confrontation. You don't have much leverage with someone you have barely met, so you're likely to lose any real battle for control.

Just as you would in any other clinical situation, remember that the patient is ill and behave accordingly. Don't use shame, guilt, or any other form of emotional blackmail. Don't plead or attempt physical restraint. If all else fails, accompany the patient as far as the door to be sure that an attendant is available, and then prepare yourself for an unusually long discussion of defense mechanisms, transference, and countertransference.

Interacting With the Examiners

After you enter the room to interview the patient, how much interaction should you have with your examiners during the next half hour? As little as possible! Your attention during this 30 minutes of information gathering should be focused exclusively on the patient. Seat yourself where you and your patient can maintain eye contact. If the examiners are completely out of your range of vision, so much the better. If you can see them, do your best to ignore them if they yawn, scratch, or take notes. (Examiners are human, too.)

Our advice to ignore examiners includes the "floater" (senior examiner) and the team leader, both of whom will pop through the door one or more times during your exam session. If you are sitting with your back to the door, you may never see who it is. That's just fine. If you keep your eyes on the patient, you run less risk of disrupting the course of your interview. If you pay attention to any of the examiners, so will your patient—at a time when you want to have the patient working for you.

On the other hand, a good time *not* to ignore examiners is when they are trying to get your attention. Although this doesn't happen frequently, examiners will sometimes see enough problems in the interview to warrant intervention. For example, a candidate could have trouble retrieving control of the interview from an unusually circumstantial patient. The examiners might try to get things back on track by saying, "Maybe you could ask about symptoms of depression."

Should your interview be interrupted that way, pay attention! The examiner isn't trying to trick or trap you, only to extract you from what may be a dead end. You would do well to take advantage of the break in the patient's monologue and respond with something like, "Yes, I was wondering that myself. Let's briefly list the symptoms of depression you have had." Even if you don't agree with the examiner's suggestion or if you feel embarrassed at being interrupted, at least make an effort to comply. This is no time to argue.

Another time you may have to shift gears suddenly is when the senior examiner drops in to check on the progress of the question-and-answer portion of an examination. Some senior examiners only observe, but others will want to ask a question or two themselves. Sometimes these questions will have been formulated on the spur of the moment by someone who hasn't heard the antecedent flow of conversation, so they may induce a sudden change of direction. Take a deep breath, relax, smile, and do your best to move in the new direction.

Chapter 6 ———————————

Taking the Psychiatric History

In format, the psychiatric Board examination interview is not much different from any other initial psychiatric interview. When you first meet any patient, you have two goals in mind. One is to establish a good working relationship. We discussed this in Chapter 5. Your other goal is to obtain the information you need to make a diagnosis, which then becomes the basis for your initial treatment plan. You have to accomplish these objectives quickly and under scrutiny, but that doesn't detract from the fact that you are about to show your competence in the clinical psychiatrist's stock-in-trade: the initial interview.

Keeping in mind that there is no single, approved method of obtaining a psychiatric history and that all histories are to some extent incomplete and inaccurate, we offer the following guide to the rapid psychiatric evaluation. If you normally do a far different type of initial interview, change your method long enough to pass this exam.

History of the Present Illness

Introductions

As soon as you are all seated together in the room and introductions have been made, thank the patient for helping with your examination and then start right in. (This is no time for irrelevant pleasantries. Remember that no one is going to quiz you later about baseball or the weather!)

From the type of facility where the examination is being held (a hospital, a clinic) you will probably know whether the patient is an outpatient or inpatient. So you can open by stating your interests explicitly. Ask:[1] "Why were you admitted here?" or "Why are you in psychiatric treatment?" A bit less directive, but still acceptable, is: "Tell me about your psychiatric problem." These opening questions state clearly where you would like to start, but at the same time leave the patient some room to maneuver. Note that this is not the time to offer your patient completely free rein. A very nondirective question such as "Where would you like to begin?" or "Tell me something about yourself" is an open-ended invitation to disaster.

Free Speech

Most authorities on interviewing advise that at first you allow the patient to talk freely about the reasons for seeking treatment. Even in an interview as time limited as this one, the practice of allowing the patient time for an opening statement is essential. For one thing, it should help the patient to relax and to confide in you. You will also get more of the flavor of personality from the patient who is allowed to talk freely than from one who is given only a rapid-fire burst of questions to answer. For another thing, free speech will give you a better understanding of your patient's main concerns. You might even be given the primary diagnosis within the first minute or two of the interview. (How much time you actually spend in each phase of the half-hour interview will depend on the patient and your own interviewing style. We discuss time elements more completely in Chapter 8, but we try to give a rough idea of the time needed for each phase of the interview in this chapter and in Chapter 7.) Free speech is also an opportunity, far in advance of the formal mental status examination, to assess the concordance of affect with the content of thought. Furthermore, during free speech you can demonstrate how well your interview style will set your patient at ease and foster rapport for the therapeutic sessions that would, in other circumstances, lie just ahead.

However, you shouldn't encourage a rambling discourse that goes nowhere. If Mrs. Riley starts to tell you about her trip last year to Sheboygan, don't wait for her to finish. You might end up knowing a great deal about her vacation and nothing at all about her depression. Instead, interrupt gently and give the open-

---

1 Throughout the next two chapters, we suggest specific questions to ask. Although we give them as direct quotations, we of course do not mean that the information must be obtained with exactly these questions. You should use an interview style that is comfortable to you and that gets the job done.

ended question another try: "You had mentioned feeling sad about that time. Could you tell me some more about that?" If this gentle prod doesn't focus the narrative sufficiently, you may have to be more direct: "Our time is short and I need to learn more about your depression. When did you start to feel bad?"

Really difficult or uncooperative patients are uncommon. Many Board examination patients are experienced interviewees, and most will be able to give a good account of themselves. The patients who volunteer for Board examinations are strongly motivated to help the candidates. They want to cooperate with you and will usually do so.

With nearly any patient you may at some point need to redirect the flow: "That was interesting about your mother, but tell me—were you depressed at other times?" Then, try to let the patient continue without interruption for another few sentences. You want an adequate sample of spontaneous speech to help you later in assessing the patient's mental status and to show your examiners that you can listen intelligently. During this phase of the interview, you should strive for an overview of the patient's problems that doesn't get lost in detail. Although some authorities on interviewing recommend that you devote up to one third of your available time to free speech, this is excessive for the brief interview necessitated by the Board exam. After 5 minutes or less (you have placed your watch where you can see it easily), you will have to move on.

Moving On to the Diagnosis

Don't ask your patient's permission to change subjects: that question is strictly pro forma, wastes time, and you don't really mean it. If the patient leaves you an opening to make a graceful transition, take it. If not, you may have to intervene more abruptly: "I think I understand some of the problems you are having. Now let me ask you about. . . ." If your patient doesn't take the hint, wait for the end of a sentence and try again: "Our time is a little short. Please tell me about. . . ." Remember that anyone can take a history from a compliant, well-organized patient. Your examiners will be very interested to learn how well you perform in more difficult interview situations.

In the free-speech phase of your interview, you will have noted clues that suggest areas to explore further. (If your patient has handed you a diagnosis on what appears to be a silver platter, examine it carefully: it may be plated!) You should spend the next 10 minutes or so developing the clues that will lead you to a diagnosis and differential diagnosis.

What sort of information will you need? Although this depends somewhat on the diagnoses you are considering, certain facts are always essential:

- Were there prior episodes of psychiatric disorder?
- When was that first episode?
- What were the possible precipitants?
- When did the patient first notice symptoms?
- When did the patient first seek treatment?
- Was there ever full recovery?

Some patients who are vague about the onset of illness may be better able to tell you when they last felt well. If you think there are two (or more) illnesses, which started first?

The history of treatment may be critically important in helping you arrive at a diagnosis quickly.

- Has the patient been hospitalized? The answer is likely to be "Yes" for Board patients.
- How many hospitalizations have there been?
- What was the overall duration?
- Does the patient know the diagnosis?
- What treatment was given?

Don't hesitate to ask questions about prior diagnoses and treatments. Anything the patient can tell you is fair game during your Board examination.

Although you will want to hear about your patient's medication history, you don't have time for a recitation of all 27 drugs that have been tried. Focus your questioning. First, if you don't already know, ask about current medicines. Try to learn the name, milligram strength, and number of doses per day of each. If your patient doesn't know the name, a description of the tablet and its side effects may help you identify it. Why was it prescribed? Don't forget to ask about electroconvulsive therapy and injectable medications.

Another potentially helpful question you can ask about drugs is, "What medicines have helped you most?" You might be surprised. The patient you thought had schizophrenia may respond, "Lithium—and I wish my doctor would prescribe it again!" Even a hospitalized patient who is currently being treated actively may tip you off to a treatment that has worked better in the past. Such information could prove valuable in the question-and-answer session later on.

As you talk with your patient, you will be roughing out the differential diagnosis in your mind. Use this time to ask questions about the symptom clusters that will allow you to rule in or out important diagnoses. Remember that the standard for diagnosis is DSM-IV, and frame your questions accordingly. If you think that your patient has bipolar mood disorder, you should be sure to identify several criteria for a manic episode. The mention of depression should trigger questions about appetite and sleep disturbances, changes of weight, diurnal variation of mood, crying spells, loss of memory and concentration, death wishes, and suicidal ideas. For each major Axis I diagnosis you plan to discuss, quickly run through the criteria to make sure that you have asked all the relevant questions.

Suicidal Behavior

Be sure to inquire about suicidal ideation and behavior. Even if there has been no hint of death wishes or suicidal ideas during the present illness, you need to ask. You can work up to the topic gradually by asking:

- Have you been having any sad, gloomy thoughts?
- Have you ever wished you were dead?
- Have you ever thought about killing yourself?
- Have you made attempts on your life?

Be sure to get details about any positive answers.

- How many attempts have you made on your life?
- Were they medically serious?
- Were they psychologically serious?
- Did they result in hospitalization?

Your questions about suicide may draw nothing but blanks, but not to ask them risks an error of omission for which an otherwise adequate examination may have trouble compensating.

Substance Use

Like suicidal behavior, drug and alcohol abuse can be found in psychiatric patients with nearly every diagnosis. Substance abuse is so common and it can so complicate the diagnostic and therapeutic picture that it must be included in every diagnostic interview. If you haven't already gathered this information, do it now. Alcohol is the most socially acceptable drug, so you might ordinarily begin with it.

Make it easy on yourself. Don't start by asking if your patient is a heavy drinker. This only invites an evasion or a value judgment—and the patient may not share your values. Instead try, "How often do you drink alcohol?" Try to get an answer in terms of days per week or per month. Next ask, "On the average day when you have at least one drink, how many drinks do you have?" And finally, "Have you ever had any problems as a result of drinking?" If necessary, specify the sorts of problems:

- Interpersonal (fights, loss of friends, guilt feelings)
- Loss of control (compulsive drinking, setting rules)
- Medical problems (vomiting, liver disorders such as jaundice, blackouts)
- Legal difficulties (including arrests and automobile accidents)
- Job problems (absence, tardiness, dismissal)
- Financial difficulties

For street drug use the drill is similar. You want to know which drugs, duration and frequency of use, and sequels. For all substances (including alcohol) you should learn whether the patient thinks there is a problem. Don't accept anyone's assertion that "I don't use drugs (alcohol) anymore." For some people, "anymore" really means "since Sunday." (Don't forget to inquire about abuse of medications prescribed by physicians, too.) If your patient has a serious problem with substance abuse, gathering this information will take some time. But you will have obtained data that have a significant bearing on the course of your patient's illness, to say nothing of your examination.

Review of Psychiatric Symptoms

Now take the time to screen for the major psychiatric symptoms and disorders that you haven't already evaluated. These include obsessions, compulsions, panic attacks, phobias, anorexia and bulimia, psychotic symptoms of hallucinations and delusions, manias, and, especially important, depression. You could save all these questions until the mental status examination, but that usually comes at the end of the interview, when time is running out. You'd be seriously embarrassed if you couldn't explore positive responses in any of these areas.

Background Information

You are now halfway through your examination, but you have obtained the basis for your diagnosis and differential diagnosis, so you have done three-fourths of your work. Now you could almost coast through the second 15 minutes with your patient, picking up details here and there and covering the balance of the material necessary for any complete medical evaluation. Actually, it will be a fairly rapid "coast," because you still must cover past medical history, a review of systems, family history, personal and social history, and the mental status evaluation.

Some of these sections will be more important for certain patients than for others. You will especially want to obtain data that might corroborate major diagnoses in your working differential: family history of depression for primary mood disorder, for example, or early truancy for a patient in whom you suspect antisocial personality disorder. You also want your examiners to understand that you realize the importance of each of these sections. Therefore, you should pace your examination so that you can at least touch on each section. However, an experienced interviewer should be able to obtain the full history as outlined here from a relatively uncomplicated patient who is a good historian.

Past Medical History

With many patients, you should be able to get through this section in a minute or two. Whereas in a complete psychiatric evaluation you might want to know the age at which your patient had measles, the rapid psychiatric evaluation simply doesn't allow time for this sort of question. Ask instead about other medications the patient may be taking. You will be especially interested in agents that could cause depression or psychosis. These include birth control pills, other hormones (such as thyroid or steroids), and antihypertensive drugs. Were diuretics prescribed for someone taking lithium? Is the patient getting psychotropic drugs from nonpsychiatric physicians?

If they haven't been mentioned previously, be sure to inquire about the emotional impact of obvious physical problems such as obesity, stuttering, a missing limb, an eye patch, or a severe limp suggesting a congenital hip dislocation. The Board examination is no time for misplaced sensitivity. Physical problems are serious enough that, if they aren't causing problems now, they probably did so at some time in the past. They will whet your examiners' curiosity, and they should whet yours, too.

Ask about medication allergies. You can acknowledge the more common ones (sulfa drugs, penicillin) with a nod of your head, but obtain a brief description of any reaction a patient has had to a psychotropic agent. Be especially careful to identify extrapyramidal side effects (akathisia, pseudoparkinsonism, acute dystonia) in patients who have been taking neuroleptics. Has there been any history suggesting tardive dyskinesia?

What about premenstrual symptoms? (They are far too often forgotten, especially by male physicians.) Have there been blackouts or other episodes that suggest a seizure disorder? What about head trauma, falls, or fainting? Does the patient receive disability benefits from Social Security, the Department of Veterans Affairs, or private insurance? A brief listing of hospitalizations for major medical illnesses and surgeries rounds out the picture of your patient's general health.

Review of Systems

No examiner can reasonably expect you to do a complete review of systems as outlined in most textbooks of medicine, but the psychiatric review of systems is our only means of reliably diagnosing somatization disorder (Briquet's syndrome), which affects about 7% of female psychiatric patients (but far less than 1% of male patients). It would be unwise to ask about *all* the DSM-IV symptoms, and simply asking whether or not a woman has enjoyed good health during her adult life has never been shown to predict the diagnosis of somatization disorder. But Othmer and DeSouza (1985) described an abbreviated screening test for somatization disorder that is quick to administer. A positive response to two or more in the following list of seven symptoms suggests a need for the complete review of systems.

The seven symptoms are

- Shortness of breath when not exerting
- Dysmenorrhea
- Burning pain in sex organs or rectum (other than with intercourse)
- Lump in throat
- Amnesia
- Vomiting
- Pain in extremities

If you don't have time to cover the complete review of systems, this checklist will at least give you some screening data in a minute or two. You can use the results later to argue the need for a full review of systems.

Family History

Although in your clinical work you might obtain a brief biographical sketch of each relative, you won't have time in the Board examination. Because a hereditary component can be identified in many psychiatric disorders, it is important to inquire about family history of psychiatric disorders. Hitting pay dirt requires careful prospecting. Ask: "Has any blood relative ever had nervousness, nervous breakdown, depression, mania, psychosis or schizophrenia, problems resulting from excessive drinking or drug abuse, suicide attempts, hypochondriasis, delinquency, legal difficulties, or hospitalization for nervousness?" (Be sure to ask slowly enough to allow your patient time to think.) Explain that by "any blood relative" you mean to include mother, father, brothers or sisters, uncles or aunts, cousins, nieces or nephews, grandparents, and children.

Remember that you cannot accept as fact an unsupported diagnosis. Your patient may not have heard the doctor correctly, or may have interpreted grandma's "spells" to mean epilepsy. Then again, one doctor's schizophrenia is another's bipolar mood disorder. Although you may not have time to mine every lode, do a little digging into the illnesses of first-degree relatives. Ask about age at onset, specific symptoms, treatment received, duration of illness, and whether the relative recovered completely or remained chronically ill. Of course, if your patient was adopted and knows nothing about any biological relatives, you should move quickly on to more fruitful inquiries.

Personal and Social History

By now you are well past the free-speech portion of your interview, and your patient should be cooperating with your increasingly structured interview style. In the typical brief interview, you will have only about 5 minutes for the personal and social history. You will be especially interested in items that have a bearing on your patient's psychiatric disorder. You will want to know how symptoms have affected the patient's life. You are also looking for events that might act as stressors—the entrances and exits of relatives and friends, for example. What changes occurred before the onset of the illness or before the current episode? Finally, your examiners will also expect you to be interested in background information that does not necessarily advance your understanding of the disease process, but only helps you get to know the patient better. Because of time constraints and the volume of information that could be developed from the personal and social history, you will have to choose carefully which questions to ask.

Childhood history. If time were no constraint, you might want to find out about your patient's formative years from open-ended questions such as, "What was it like growing up in Newark during the War?" Unfortunately, you don't have time to indulge in that luxury. Because the answers will little enhance your prospects either for diagnosis or for rapport with the patient, you should avoid certain questions that you might ask in a more extended interview This is especially true of many events from early childhood, some of which tend to be neither relevant nor reliably reported. So put aside any questions you usually ask about the patient's gestation, delivery, birth weight, breast-feeding, toilet training, and other developmental milestones. Concentrate on material you can expect to benefit from. For the sake of this discussion, let us assume you are interviewing a man.

You want to know how many siblings he had and what his position was in that sibship. What was his father's occupation? Did his mother work outside the home? Was he reared by both parents? Were there any divorces or deaths in the family? How far did he go in school, and how well did he do academically? Did he have disciplinary problems in school? Did he attend religious services as a child? Did this change when he grew up? Was he sickly as a child, and did he receive any rewards (secondary gain) for illness behavior?

Job history. What is your patient's occupation, and how long has he held his current job? If his current employment has been brief, how many jobs has he held in the last 5 years? If he is unemployed, why? What has been the effect of illness on his job performance? If he does not support himself by working, what is his source of income?

Military history. (Although we are still talking about a theoretical male patient, remember that military history can apply to women as well. The Board examination is no time to appear sexist.) How long did the patient serve in the military? In what branch (Air Force, Army, Coast Guard, Marines, Navy)? What was the highest rank he attained? Were there disciplinary problems (captain's mast, court martial, company grade punishment, Article 15)? What kind of discharge did he receive?

Legal history. When you covered alcohol-related offenses such as driving while intoxicated or arrests for public drunkenness, you may have asked about general legal difficulties. If not, do so now. Has the patient ever been arrested? How many times? On what charges? Has he been jailed? Did he ever serve time in the penitentiary? How long was he there?

Marital and sexual history. You probably learned much earlier whether or not your patient is currently married. But is this his first marriage? If he is divorced, find out why. How old was he when first married? How long has the current marriage lasted? Are there children or stepchildren? Has psychiatric illness impaired the patient's marital relationship or ability to care for his family?

Your discussion of marriage(s) provides a natural lead-in to questions about sexual satisfaction and practices. Does the couple use birth control? Have there been severe problems with intercourse, perhaps requiring abstinence? Does the patient experience satisfactory climax with intercourse? Has there been impotence? Have there been sex partners outside the current relationship? Try to get the patient to describe sexual dysfunctions and practices in behavioral terms: "First I . . . then she does . . . then this happens. . . ."

Even unmarried patients and adolescents should be asked about their sexual activities. Be particularly alert for evidence of multiple sexual partners, homosexuality, and other behaviors that predict exposure to the AIDS virus. Have high-risk patients been tested for HIV? Do they always use condoms?

Now would be a good time to inquire about childhood sexual molestation. Although this is a factor in the histories of 20% or more of psychiatric patients, few psychiatrists routinely obtain this information. Try to get details. What acts occurred and at what ages? Was there physical contact? Who perpetrated the acts? Was incest involved? Did the parents find out? How did they respond? How was the patient affected?

Religion. At some point, you should ask about religion. With which (if any) religion does your patient identify? Is it the same as it was during childhood? How devout is your patient? In addition to the literal responses, you may hear some ideas on the meaning of life or what organizes the universe, developed at the patient's own cognitive level.

Social relationships. All patients, including those most isolated in the back wards of a chronic facility, are social beings. The information they report to their physicians is influenced by past and current relationships. As you go through the historical items we have discussed in this chapter, you should also be forming a picture of your patient's social interactions and milieus at different times of life.

This picture will usually start with the household where the patient grew up. Your understanding of the patient's personality development may be enhanced by information about childhood relationships with parents, siblings, other relatives in the household, neighbors, and friends. You will be better able to discuss Axis II disorders, prognosis, and the indications for psychotherapy if you have learned something about your patient's relationships (and conflicts) in the current household, network of social support, and opportunities for communication. A therapeutic formulation should take into account those persons who are likely to help or interfere with treatment. You will want to know who among them will need better information or a different point of view to promote the patient's well-being.

You will be interested in knowing something about your patient's personality and leisure activities. Time permitting, you might ask: "What sort of a person do you think are you? Have you been outgoing or a loner? What do you like about yourself? What do your friends like about you? What do you do for fun?"

Finally, although you probably learned it long ago, do you know how old your patient is now? Better to ask late than never!

Chapter 7 —————————————————————

Mental Status Examination

Originally, the mental status examination (MSE) was an amplified part of the neurological exam. Today, it is fundamental to the workup of any patient, psychiatric or otherwise. It should be no less an integral part of the monitored examination. Although occasionally you may be able to assess the patient adequately without a formal MSE, it may be 1) hard to identify that rare patient and 2) less trouble to go ahead and do an MSE than to defend not doing one. However, one examiner points out that candidates are sometimes asked to justify asking about certain items of history or performing a formal MSE when the clinical picture doesn't warrant it. We maintain that this task is infinitely easier than explaining why you didn't ask when you should have.

By now, only about 5 minutes are probably left in your patient interview. If you are like many other candidates, you may be tempted to ignore the MSE as you struggle to extract every last drop of history. Although for many patients you can omit portions of the formal MSE, the structure of the Board examinations requires that each candidate demonstrate skill at administering and evaluating it.

What Is Most Important in the Mental Status Examination?

Not every patient will require the same attention to the MSE. You probably won't be able to complete it, and your examiners don't expect you to do so. With time short, they want to know how well you can focus on what is most important for you to understand your patient. Therefore, your key question is, "Under what circumstances should I do a more thorough MSE?" For most patients you might

75

encounter during the Boards, you will have to choose portions of the formal MSE that are most likely to yield important data. That will require judgment on your part, but you can rely on several guiding principles:

1. Several parts of the MSE come "for free." To learn about them, you don't have to ask anything special; just pay attention while you are taking the history and you will be able to report on the patient's general appearance and behavior, the flow of thought, and portions of the sensorium.
2. Watch for behavior that suggests specific deficits. Repetitive physical actions should alert you to the possibility of obsessions; motor restlessness may be due to akathisia, which would suggest that you probe the content of thought for delusions and hallucinations.
3. Listen to what your patient tells you. For example, a history of head injury or seizures demands that you pay more attention to the details of the sensorium such as memory. If the patient reports hallucinations, do ask carefully about delusions as well.
4. Certain diagnoses in your differential require more careful testing of the sensorium. Alcoholism and dementia are two obvious examples.
5. Certain parts of the MSE should be included for nearly any patient you might encounter during the Boards. These essentials include questions about mood, suicide, and psychosis. You should be able to describe the three dimensions that characterize your patient's affect.

You should consider doing a fuller MSE for older patients (geriatric age range) and for those who have intercurrent medical disease. In particular, the suspicion of AIDS should evoke more attention to the sensorium.

The Traditional Mental Status Examination

The MSE is traditionally divided into six parts; psychiatrists traditionally differ as to the order, emphasis, and content of the parts. Which form of the MSE you use matters less than the fact that you use one at all. To ensure that you evaluate and describe every aspect of each patient's mental status, you should choose an MSE format that you are comfortable with, memorize the parts in that order, and apply that format rigorously to each patient you interview.

The following is one such format that has stood the test of time. In describing it, we will try to define briefly all the terms you need to know. But again, we emphasize that no candidate will be expected to use the complete MSE as we have outlined it here. Be sure you know it all, but choose those parts you need to evaluate your own Board patient.

I. General Appearance and Behavior

A great deal of the MSE can (and should) be done by observation alone. In that way, your senses do double duty: you gather information visually and verbally at the same time. When candidates forget this, they can come to grief.

> When Dr. Voner entered the room, the patient was already seated quietly, fore-head covered by slightly unkempt hair. So the bullet hole scar in the forehead went unnoticed. When the patient left the room, the candidate (who was busy taking notes) also missed the slight limp. Observing these two physical conditions could have made a real difference in the quality of Dr. Voner's life during the next half hour. As it was, after the patient had departed, the examiners themselves had to point out these physical signs and suggest that the patient had shot himself, producing a hemiparesis and a partial lobotomy.

Your observations of appearance and behavior begin the moment you meet your patient. (We'll continue to discuss our hypothetical male patient.) Does he walk with a limp? Does he shake hands when you greet one another? Is his grip firm? Are his hands dry or clammy? Does he appear to be his stated age? How would you describe his general condition? Well nourished? Unshaven? Tousled? Malodorous? Is his clothing clean or dirty, fashionable or out of date? Does the clothing fit the climate? Is he responsive, alert, and cooperative, or does he refuse eye contact, turn away, and sulk? Notice any unusual motor activity: Is he over-active or underactive? Is he stuporous (unresponsive without being asleep)? Is he restless? Does he pick at his skin or clothes?

Notice his speech. Is it accented? Does he stutter? Does his voice have a normal lilt? (This is called *prosody*.)

He may show *mannerisms* (unnecessary behavior that is part of a goal-directed act, such as the introductory flourish some people make with a pen as they start to write) or *stereotypies* (non-goal-directed behavior, such as making the sign of the cross every second sentence or so). Is there evidence of *posturing* (striking a pose and maintaining it)? *Waxy flexibility* (resistance of limbs to passive motion, like bending a wax rod or lead pipe)? *Catalepsy* (maintaining any position, no matter how uncomfortable, for a period of time)?

Look closely for signs of extrapyramidal side effects that might indicate the use of neuroleptic drugs. Extrapyramidal side effects include *pseudoparkinsonism* (masklike face, pill-rolling tremor, and general muscular rigidity) and *akathisia* (the need to get up or pace around the room). You are unlikely to encounter a fourth extrapyramidal side effect, *acute dystonia*, during this examination. You could conceivably encounter *tardive dyskinesia* as well, but this might be manifested only by subtle signs such as tongue fasciculations. At any rate, you should be prepared to discuss this tragic side effect of medication.

II. *Affect*

Many psychiatrists maintain that there is a difference between *mood* and *affect*. Unfortunately, they cannot always agree as to what that difference is. Some define *affect* as a transient state of feeling and *mood* as a feeling of longer duration. Some define the terms as just the opposite. In another system, mood describes a person's subjective feeling and affect describes how the person appears to be feeling. According to the latter system of definition, affect would include downcast eyes, the slope of the shoulders, and the droop of the lip. More and more, the terms *mood* and *affect* are used interchangeably. Use them as you will, but be able to defend your usage and remember that some psychiatrists still insist on the distinction.

Too often physicians content themselves with a one- or two-word description of mood (affect): "Seems depressed" or "Flat affect." An adequate description always includes three parameters: type, lability, and appropriateness.

Type of affect.   Is the patient's overall affect one of depression, anxiety, fear, irritability, euphoria, or hostility? "About medium" or "normal in type" will do as a description, if the patient's affect is unremarkable. Two affects may sometimes coexist: a manic patient may show euphoria and irritability almost at the same time. (During any given half hour, even psychiatrically normal people may show more than one affect.) However, you probably won't have the time to discover your patient's full range of affect. You will have to make do with the dominant affect(s) you detect during your interview.

Lability of affect.   Does the patient's affect remain stable, or does it change noticeably during your interview? Some degree of affective lability is normal; when it is absent, we call it *blunting* or *flattening* of affect. Schizophrenia patients sometimes have blunted affect, but it is by no means diagnostic: it can also be found in severe depression and in Parkinson's disease, to name just two. *Increased lability* of affect is sometimes encountered in somatization disorder (also know as Briquet's syndrome, or hysteria) and in dementia. When severe, as in dementias, excessive lability of affect is sometimes termed *affective incontinence*.

Appropriateness of affect.   Of necessity, characterizing appropriateness of affect is highly subjective. You attempt to state whether or not the patient's affect matches the situation and the content of the patient's own thought. The patient who laughs while recounting his mother's death or screams obscenities during introductions may be said to have *inappropriate affect*. In somatization disorder, you may occasionally encounter the special type of inappropriate affect termed *la belle indifférence* (lofty indifference). It means that your patient regards serious symptoms such as paralysis or blindness, which would severely upset most people, with a bland lack of concern.

III. Flow of Thought

Of course, what we really mean is *flow of speech,* but we assume that patterns of thought are mirrored in the patient's speech. Flow of thought includes 1) disturbances of association (the way in which syllables and words are strung together in phrases and sentences and the relationship of the patient's answers to the questions) and 2) disturbances of the rate and rhythm of speech. These divisions are somewhat arbitrary, and the boundaries are often blurred. We will, therefore, present them all together. (We have adapted the following discussion from Andreasen 1979a and 1979b.)

In *circumstantial speech,* the patient includes many trivial and unnecessary details, but the connection between ideas is clear and the point is eventually made. In *distractible speech,* the patient's attention may be diverted by an extraneous stimulus (a noise or movement from one of your examiners could stop your patient in midthought).

Derailment is a pattern of spontaneous speech in which one idea runs into another that may be related clearly, if incompletely, or into one that bears no apparent relationship at all. The sequence of ideas can be understood, but the direction changes often and the succession of ideas may be governed less by logic than by rhyming, punning, or other associations that may have meaning for the patient, but not for the observer.

This term replaces several others that once were thought to carry some additional diagnostic meaning but are now generally acknowledged to be unreliable. One of these, *flight of ideas,* is usually accompanied by pressured speech (see below) and has always been linked with mania. It implies that the speaker moves rapidly from one idea to the next. Another is *loose associations,* which is a generic term for thoughts that do not hang together logically. This term has classically been linked with schizophrenia. The preferred term *derailment* carries no implication of diagnosis.

> When asked how long he had been hospitalized, a manic patient responded, "I've been here a week, I was weak when they admitted me, that's quite an admission to make, don't you think?"

Tangentiality, also called tangential speech, is a term that should be used only to describe an answer to a question. The answer may seem utterly irrelevant to the question, or there may be some vague or distant relationship.

CANDIDATE.   How are you feeling today, Mrs. Jordan?
MRS. JORDAN.   Are you my father?
CANDIDATE.   I don't think I understood that.
MRS. JORDAN.   I've got bricks in my bats.

A number of other association patterns of speech occur much less often than those just mentioned. The dictionary is crammed with words and phrases used to describe them all. Some of those could come up in the context of discussing your patient (or the videotape) with the examiners. We'll review some of the more common ones.

The term *stilted speech* applies to a patient who, for example, affects a British accent (without being British) or uses quaint or out-of-fashion phrases. The patient who *perseverates* repeats the same idea (sentence, phrase, word) over and over again, despite your attempts to channel the conversation elsewhere. (Constant repetition of isolated words is sometimes called *verbigeration*.) *Echolalia* occurs when the patient slavishly repeats the words or statements of others. When a word is invented by connecting syllables in novel ways, it is called a *neologism. Incoherence,* a speech pattern that the average listener cannot comprehend, may be due to use of random words *(word salad)* or to the suspension of the usual rules of grammar. Be careful not to overdiagnose incoherence, especially when it may be due to neurological disorders or to the speech patterns of a person whose native language is not English.

Clang association occurs when words are strung together solely on the basis of a similar sound (How now, brown cow). Word associations may also show *alliteration,* in which stressed syllables have similar sounds.

> Mr. Future, a patient in Leo Rosten's novel *Captain Newman, M.D.*, uses alliterative speech: "One encounters similar contretemps with the cluttering, clamorous clods in the unmedical corps upstairs. . . ."

Push of speech refers to an increased amount of speech that is usually rapid and is often loud and difficult to interrupt. It may be accompanied by *decreased latency of response,* in which the answer is given almost before you finish your question. Although it is characteristic of mania, it can be found in other pathological conditions as well as in a few otherwise normal individuals who simply talk too fast and too much. In an examination situation, you may find yourself continually having to pull on the reins to keep control of the patient who has one of these speech patterns.

On the other hand, a depressed patient may have *poverty of speech* (a reduction in the amount of spontaneous speech). Replies may be brief or monosyllabic when elaboration of a thought is clearly called for, or speech may be offered only in response to questions. In either event, you must do more than your share of the work of the interview. You could also encounter an *increased latency of response,* in which the patient takes longer than normal to answer a question. *Blocking* occurs when speech suddenly stops, interrupting a thought sequence. *Mutism,* in which the patient does not attempt to speak at all yet presumably retains the ability to do so, should be distinguished from *aphonia,* in which the patient can only whisper or speak in a hoarse croak. The former is a more serious psychiatric symptom. The latter may have medical or neurological implications, but it may also be associated with somatoform disorders.

IV. Content of Thought

By this point in your mental status examination, you might feel tempted to cut some corners. Avoid the temptation: you must have some of this information, and your examiners will ask you about some of it.

Of all the parts of the MSE, *suicidal ideation* is perhaps the least expendable. It should be touched on by direct questioning in every patient, regardless of the suspected diagnosis. In Chapter 6, we covered the sorts of questions you should ask relevant to a history of suicidal behavior. You also must learn whether the patient is having any such thoughts now. A positive answers demands appropriate follow-up questions:

- How long has the patient entertained these thoughts?
- How serious are they now?
- Is there a current plan for suicide?
- Is there a timetable?
- Does the patient have the means to commit suicide?

Selection for your examination does not mean that your patient is certified as being free of suicidal ideas. In fact, more than once a Board examination candidate has uncovered serious psychopathology that was previously unsuspected.

Just as serious, though far less common, are *homicidal thoughts.* These ideas, plus ideas about committing other acts of violence, should always be pursued. This is especially true when the patient has admitted to a history of violent behavior or feelings of uncontrollable rage.

Phobias are intense, unreasonable fears associated with some situation or object. Psychiatrists used to stock a whole lexicon of named phobias that today seems a useless exercise in semantics. (Who cares that *siderodromophobia* means fear of travel by railroad?) *Acrophobia* (fear of heights), *claustrophobia* (fear of being closed in), and *agoraphobia* (fear of open places or of being away from home) occur commonly enough that the names are still useful. Ascertain duration (recent versus long term) and intensity (does the phobia interfere with usual activities?).

An *obsession* is a thought, idea, or belief that dominates thought content and persists despite the person's recognition that it is unrealistic or senseless. *Compulsions* are the motor counterpart of obsessions. They often result in repetitive rituals that significantly interfere with the person's activities of daily living. A defining feature of obsessions and compulsions is the patient's desire to resist them. Ask, "Have you had any thoughts that seem silly, but that you keep thinking over and over? Are there any rituals that you cannot seem to resist?" Ascertain duration and intensity as for phobias.

Hallucinations are false sensory perceptions occurring in the absence of a related external sensory stimulus. Hallucinations can be graded as to severity. For example, auditory hallucinations, the most common, could be categorized progressively as indistinct noises, mumbling, distinct words, phrases, and sentences. Many patients will understand what you mean if you simply ask, "Do you hear voices?" But people who don't hallucinate (and some who do hallucinate but who have less experience in talking with psychiatrists) may think you meant to say, "Can you hear a person's voice when you are being spoken to?" To avoid time-consuming ambiguity on this point, always ask, "Do you hear voices when there is no one around?"

Expand on positive answers by asking, "Are these voices as clear to you as my voice is now?" Ascertain location: for auditory hallucinations, do they come from within the patient's head or body, from out in the hall, or from a specific source such as the cocker spaniel or grandma's crazy quilt? How often do they occur? How does the patient explain them? (Part of an illness? Alien influence?) How does the patient react to them? (Bemusement? Fear? Obedience?) *Audible thoughts* (the experience of hearing one's own thoughts spoken aloud) are a special form of auditory hallucination; it has similar import.

Visual hallucinations are much less often encountered but may be graded progressively as flashes of light, indistinct images, fully formed people, scenes, and tableaux. The tactile hallucination of ants crawling on or beneath the skin is called *formication*. Olfactory and gustatory hallucinations occur infrequently and may indicate a delirium with psychosis.

Illusions are misinterpretations of actual sensory stimuli. They usually occur in the context of limited sensory stimulation (such as low light) and are normal—nearly everyone has had the experience of awakening at night and being momentarily afraid of attack, perhaps from the dim form of a bathrobe thrown across the back of a chair. A patient who has had an illusion will sometimes require the reassurance that it is not the same as "going crazy"; this reassurance may be given freely, if quickly.

A *delusion* is a fixed, false belief not explained by the patient's culture and education. Ask: "Have you felt that anyone was spying on you, following you, or trying to read your thoughts or influence you in some way?" *Fixed* is a key word. Before a patient's statement that "someone has parked a frankfurter in my ear" is marked down as a delusion, it must first be distinguished from an "as if" experience.

CANDIDATE.   Do you really believe that?
PATIENT.   Well, it hurts as much as if someone had put a frankfurter there!

The patient's response shows that he may accept another interpretation of his experience. Thus, it is not a delusion. Occasionally, a patient may say something that sounds delusional, but is really not. The high-powered industrial tycoon who agrees (perhaps partly in jest) that he is God may be an example. A patient may either uncritically accept a delusion but realize that other people disbelieve it or may expect the same uncritical acceptance of others.

Delusions also come in a variety of styles and colors. They can be circumscribed, involving one or several areas of thought and behavior, or massive, occupying nearly all of the patient's energy. A *delusional system* incorporates many life experiences that the patient interprets as a part of the central (usually persecutory) idea.

If your patient has *persecutory* delusions, he believes that he is being ridiculed, deliberately interfered with, discriminated against, spied on, or threatened. He usually believes that these indignities are undeserved, but if he also has delusions of *guilt* he may feel that they are retribution for his sins and that he deserves them. He may believe that his actions or thoughts are being controlled or influenced in an unusual way, such as by radio waves, television, or witchcraft: these are delusions of *passivity or influence*. He may claim to "know" that people are talking about, spying on, or slandering him: these are delusions of *reference*. This type of delusion may be confirmed when the patient "sees" others turn their heads and whisper as he walks by. Television, radio programs, or the newspapers may contain messages that are meant explicitly for him. If severely depressed, the patient may develop delusions of *ill health or bodily change*, believing, for example, that he has syphilis, he is becoming insane, his bowels have petrified, his brain is rotting, his genitals have shrunk, and so on. If he has delusions of *jealously*, he may believe that his partner has been unfaithful. Delusions of jealousy are typical of alcoholism, but are not confined to it. If your patient has delusions of *grandeur*, he believes that he is a person of some exalted station or has powers not accorded ordinary mortals.

Several other types of psychopathology should be distinguished from delusions. *Depersonalization* is the persistent feeling that the individual has changed, whereas *derealization* refers to the similar feeling that the environment has changed. Déjà vu (French for "already seen") is the feeling of having seen or experienced a particular situation before, when that is probably not the case. Déjà vu is normal. *Overvalued ideas* are beliefs that are maintained in contradiction to their evident worth. Examples are the inherent superiority of one's sex, race, political party, or school of psychotherapy.

V. *Sensorium and Intellectual Resources*

Orientation.   From the beginning of your interview, it should be obvious whether your patient—let's call him Mr. Johnson—knows his own name (is oriented to person). No one will fault you for not asking this question. But, although it is true that an experienced psychiatrist in everyday practice often does not ask a patient to respond to other questions on orientation, the Board exam is far from everyday. You had better find out whether your patient can tell the date (within a day or two) and place (the name of the town, the name of the building or what kind of institution you are in). At the outset of this phase of the MSE, you can lessen your discomfort at the pursuit of such obvious subjects by admitting, "Psychiatrists ask a lot of obvious questions. Now I'd like to ask you a few of these routine questions." When interpreting deficiencies, consider the possibility of impaired memory or motivation as alternative explanations.

Memory.   Memory is usually divided into three parts. Most of it can be assessed without elaborate testing. You can best judge recent memory from your patient's ability to organize recent events into their proper sequence as the history of the present illness unfolds. It is traditional to test memory by asking questions such as, "What did you have for breakfast?" or "When were you married?" But because in the Board examination you cannot validate the accuracy of the response, you are probably better off not following the routine you use in your clinical practice. You might ask, "How long have you had to wait?"—which at least should be immediately verifiable. If the patient drove to the exam site, you could ask where the car is parked—which you could also verify quickly.

A test of *retention and recall* requires a little more effort, but it provides a verifiable test of memory. State a color, a person's name, and a street address. Ask for an immediate repetition to be sure the patient has heard and understood, but don't give a warning that you will ask for another repetition later (this would invite rehearsal). After 5 minutes, ask for a recitation of the items as you presented them. Be sure to take into consideration the patient's motivation when you interpret the results of this test. If you wish, lead into these questions by saying, "Have you had any problems with your memory? I'd like to ask a few questions to test it." Warning: if you use this test, be sure you remember to ask about the three items later.

Calculations. Have the patient subtract 7 from 100 and continue to subtract 7 from each successive answer. Most adults make fewer than four errors and finish within 60 seconds, but two or three successive (and successful) subtractions will probably suffice. If serial 7s are too hard, try serial 3s subtracted from 20. Can the patient do simple multiplication? As an alternative task, ask for simple, serial multiplications: $2 \times 3 = 6$, $2 \times 6 = 12$, ... $2 \times 48 = 96$. The ability to complete this task without error correlates strongly with an IQ of 85 or better. Maxmen (1986) suggested that asking your patient to count backward by 1s from (say) 57, stopping at 42, is a less culture-bound test of attention and concentration, which is what you are really trying to evaluate by asking for calculations.

Ability with calculations must be correlated (in your presentation after the patient leaves the room) with age, culture, and education. Even when the patient is obviously bright and mathematically adept, for the sake of completeness you should probably ask for a few calculations.

General information. From your previous 25 minutes of conversation, you probably already have a good indication of what your patient knows, especially if politics, sports, and other items of current interest have come up in the course of history taking. If not, here is another portion of the MSE where you must demonstrate competence. Ask: "Who is President of the United States now? Who served just before?" Most adults can name the past five presidents in order, beginning with the current one. Other similar tests you will rarely need include the following: Name the governor of the state. Name five large cities or five rivers. In interpreting results, consider the patient's anxiety, depression, sensorium, education, motivation, and degree of political interest.

Abstractions. Inability to abstract general meaning from a proverb was once regarded as characteristic of schizophrenia. Research data have long since demonstrated that the facility for this sort of mental activity has far more to do with education, culture, and native intelligence than with sanity. How well your patient, Mr. Johnson, was able to formulate the problem that brought him into treatment should by this time have given you plenty of information about his ability to make abstractions. But if you have time to spare, you could ask: "What does it mean when I say, 'People who live in glass houses shouldn't throw stones?' " The answer "They might break windows" is a *concrete* sort of interpretation that indicates poor abstracting ability. (Note that "A rolling stone gathers no moss" commonly elicits one of two opposite, but equally valid, interpretations.)

Other, less culture-bound tasks of abstraction include the ability to tell similarities ("How are an apple and an orange alike?"—both are fruits, round, have seeds, etc.) and differences ("What's the difference between a child and a dwarf?"—the child will grow). Many clinicians prefer similarities to proverbs as a test of abstracting ability.

With time to kill, a psychiatrist will sometimes try to learn whether a patient can identify verbal absurdities, as in the butcher story: "One day while dressing meat, a butcher accidentally cut his hand off. This made him so angry he picked up the cleaver and cut his other hand off." However, if you have this much time to spare, you may well have missed something vital in your patient's history. Don't fiddle; Rome is burning.

VI. *Insight and Judgment*

Insight means that Mr. Johnson realizes he is ill (if this is the case) and that he understands something about the nature of that illness. In the context of the MSE, insight does not refer to putative etiologic or psychodynamic aspects of illness. If you don't already have a good assessment of insight, ask the following sort of question: "What problems do you have?" or "Are you sick in any way?" or "What kind of sickness do people have here (in the clinic or hospital)?"

Judgment is sometimes tested by asking how the patient would respond to finding a stamped letter on the ground or discovering a fire in a crowded theater. The answer might give you some idea of the patient's ability to deal with correspondence or conflagrations, but this does not necessarily reflect an ability to cope in the real world. Judgment is better assessed by history from an informant, but the structure of the Board examination makes this impossible. However, you may be able to infer judgment from your patient's statements about any previous treatment. If not, ask: "What are your plans for the near future?" or "How does your future look to you?" or "Do you think you need treatment?"

Chapter 8 ————————————————

The 30-Minute Hour

Performing a thorough psychiatric interview under the pressure of time is stressful at best, yet many psychiatrists do it every day. When you do a brief interview in routine practice, it is usually by choice. If you have a difficult office patient, you can always choose to spend more time interviewing and less time eating lunch.

Board candidates, with no discretionary time available, not only must perform a creditable exam in 30 minutes flat, but also must do it under the scrutiny of strangers. So it is no wonder that even as they introduce themselves, candidates typically feel they are about to run out of time. In this chapter, we discuss how you can best make use of the half hour allotted to examining a patient during the Board examinations.

Time Management

Watch the Clock

You can't manage time if you don't know how much of it you have left, and the examination room is almost certain to have no clock readily visible. Be sure to ask the examiners to give you a 5-minute warning. Place your wristwatch on the table in front of you where you can see it easily. This lacks elegance, but it beats having to steal a surreptitious glance at your wrist every few minutes, and it is vastly superior to being caught with half your interview to go and only 5 minutes remaining.

You won't learn what time you are to begin your patient interview until you register for the exam, so you won't know whether it will begin on the half hour or at some other odd time (see Chapter 4 for time schedules). The actual patient exam is stressful enough that you shouldn't use your energy mentally subtracting minutes from, say, 10 or 50 minutes past the hour to see how much time you have left. Instead, you might consider using a stopwatch, or resetting your wristwatch so that 12 o'clock coincides with the start of your patient interview (an electronic watch with a dual time feature should work well). That way, you can concentrate on the patient's information without having to perform serial mental arithmetic of your own.

When you enter the room, you should know about how many minutes you will spend on each part of the examination. (See Chapters 6 and 7 for a more complete description of the different phases of the examination.) Of course, how you divide your time will vary with the individual patient, but as a general rule you should plan as follows:

- 5 minutes: Chief complaint and free speech
- 7 minutes: Specific questions to rule diagnoses in or out, elicit pertinent negatives, and inquire about suicidal ideas, violence, alcohol and drug history
- 5 minutes: Medical history, review of systems, family history
- 5 minutes: Personal and social history, evaluation of character pathology
- 5 minutes: Mental status examination
- 3 minutes: Buffer time to catch up on last questions and pursue other late-developing leads

In practice, most interviews are probably shaded toward more time to elaborate the present illness. But even if you don't stick to it strictly, an approximate timetable will help you to touch on all the critical points. In any event, these times may vary widely, depending on the characteristics of your patient.

"Hard" and "Easy" Patients

Board exam patients certainly can present a variety of challenges. Your patient may cause you some anxious moments with one or more of the following characteristics:

- Vague history (probably the most common attribute)
- Circumstantial speech
- Difficult-to-understand speech (actually, patients who speak in unfamiliar accents may be more of a problem for repeating candidates; first timers will usually be examined in their own part of the country)

- Suspiciousness or hostility
- Complicated history

Any one of these attributes can cause problems in a half-hour exam. Combine several, as happens often, and you will face an exacting test of your ability to forge rapport while managing the interview.

Actually, you should expect that most patients will have some quirk of personality or mental status that will tax your interviewing skills. After all, most of these people have sought treatment because of emotional or interpersonal difficulties. You cannot expect them to recite their life stories as if written up in a textbook. In this sense, there is no such thing as a bad patient—only those who present with different sorts of challenges to overcome. If the patient presents some difficulty in the interview, don't regard it as a calamity. Remember that you'll have far more opportunity to show your skill with a difficult patient than with an easy one.

Still, if your patient is intelligent, alert, and observant and can tell a coherent story that is to the point, you'll probably breathe a little easier. Although you should never try to let your patient do the work for you, an easy patient can certainly brighten your day at the Boards. But if you rely on such extraordinary luck, the consequences could be dire. Take a pointer from the disaster-planning experts: hope for the best but plan for the worst.

Develop Rapport If You Can

The word *If* is critical. You should certainly try to establish a good working relationship with your patient (see Chapter 5). But the need for rapport is relative. Although you would like to have both rapport and a complete history, the latter is more important by far. Theoretically, you could successfully negotiate the Boards with no rapport at all (as long as you showed that you tried to form a relationship with your patient), but not without information.

Of course, if you can develop a friendly working relationship, you'll get your patient's best efforts at cooperation, and that could mean you will get more information in less time. So make the effort to achieve a good working relationship, but make it quickly.

You may be able to win some sympathy if at the beginning you remind your patient that you are being tested and that you appreciate the cooperation. Establish eye contact early in the interview and continue it throughout, but avoid fixed stares. A nod or smile conveys your empathy and silently reassures the patient, "You're doing fine." (This maneuver takes no time, yet shows the examiners that you, too, are doing fine.) Be responsive and sympathetic to both the content of the history and to the patient's affect.

Your patient will probably relax and talk more freely if you seem at ease yourself. If you have to fake an air of relaxation, then do so. (Some candidates have obtained good results by practicing in front of a mirror.) Of course, your best bet for achieving good rapport is to be genuinely interested in the story your patient has to tell.

You'll definitely look and feel more relaxed if you are not madly taking notes throughout the interview. Instead, during the interview mentally organize the information you obtain and file it away (in your head) under sections of the standard interview format (see Chapter 6). Mentally note the specific information you want to emphasize during your presentation, and try to get a sense of your own feelings about the patient.

Controlling the Interview

You must be in charge of the interview, even if you have to be more firm than usual. In the most favorable case, being firm may mean nothing more than interjecting an occasional gentle question to guide the progress of the interview. But you should be prepared, after the first few minutes of free speech, to become hard-nosed and insistent if the interview begins to go awry.

Most patients won't try too hard to be controlling. Treated for years in teaching facilities, many patients have been interviewed by numerous physicians and other mental health professionals at all levels of training. They know quite well how to cooperate with an interview. Still, you could encounter a patient with a thirst for control, evidenced by manic pressure of speech, psychotic suspiciousness of your motives, or overall normal appearance but circumstantial manner. You would then have to take steps to keep your entire interview from being ruined.

Structure is the key to your success. Although you may not exactly follow the timetable you have in mind, it should remind you to cover many categories of information in your half hour. Even though you have not plumbed every depth in the psychiatric history, you must keep moving and touch on everything.

After the first few minutes, you must stop asking open-ended questions. This strategy may go considerably against the grain; however, once you know the general outline of your patient's problems, you should be able to frame a number of short-answer questions that will allow you to test and discard successive hypotheses as to diagnosis.

You won't have time to respond as completely as you would like to your patient's expressed emotion. But you can show your interest while getting further information by asking, for example, "When have you felt depressed like this before?" If your patient seems troubled by a recent problem that you have already explored, you could say something like, "I'd like to hear more about that later if we have time. Now we must move on." Periodically, you may have to reinforce your expectation of concise, informative answers. You may find yourself having to cut short attempts to expand on yes or no answers when the extra verbiage doesn't materially advance your progress. If the patient gets off the track, use variations on "We only have a few minutes" or "Now I'd like to ask you some short-answer questions."

It helps to remember that the purpose of this interview is diagnostic, not therapeutic. It isn't your job to practice nondirective psychotherapy, to give advice, or to inspect skin lesions or pictures of grandchildren. If the patient improves as a result of your talk, that's well and good, but your only real task is to pass the exam. Don't offer therapeutic recommendations to the patient, who is, after all, not *your* patient. Whatever else, don't be like one candidate who lectured an adolescent patient on morals.

No matter what you think of the present treatment plan, don't criticize it to the patient. In fact, if you make any treatment recommendations, you risk inducing mistrust of the patient's own physician. Also, you would put yourself in the impossible position of claiming some responsibility for a patient you don't know well and will never see again. Neither should you offer false reassurance; if your patient asks for help of some sort, respond with something on the order of: "Your own doctor knows you better and can give you the best advice on this." Interpretations are none of your business, either, even if you have time.

In any first interview, some topics are of little use. From such topics you are unlikely to obtain information valuable enough to justify the time spent in asking. Toilet training is one such topic; others include developmental milestones and childhood diseases. (Few adults can reliably tell you the age at which they first walked or spoke sentences, anyway.) Don't discuss dreams, even if they are offered. In the 30-minute interview, dreams are the royal road to oblivion. Keep practicing interview control: "I'd love to know that, but first. . . ." "I really need to hear about. . . ." "Our time is running short."

Always keep a tight rein on your own verbal output. Two important principles apply. 1) Anxiety may cause you to talk more freely than you normally do. 2) The more time you spend talking, the less time your patient will have to give you information. Formulate your questions as clearly and succinctly as you can. Save your opinions, complaints, and comments for later. You'll be given your own free speech time after the patient leaves the room.

Red Flags

Before we leave the subject of time management, here's another word of warning: Be alert for "red flags." These are unexpected bits of information that warn you of areas you need to explore. Red flags can pop up any time, but they are most likely to take you unaware when you have obtained most of your history and are trying to tie up loose ends with some short-answer questions.

Here's an example: You've sailed smoothly through a history of what sounds like straightforward schizophrenia. After mopping up a last few items of family history, you're almost ready for the formal part of your mental status exam.

YOU: Mr. Carson, has anyone else in your family ever had a psychiatric illness?
PATIENT: No one except my sister. She was hospitalized for awhile just before my first blackout.

First blackout? This is the first you've heard about *any* blackouts, and you're almost at the end of the exam! What does he mean by blackouts, anyway? Seizures? (He's already denied any other health problems.) Alcoholic blackouts? (You're almost sure he doesn't drink heavily.)

What a predicament. His sister's illness might help nail down a diagnosis of schizophrenia, but you also have to follow up on his blackouts. They could have real bearing on why he is psychotic. And time is rapidly running out.

No problem. You have time—that's why you have the 3 minutes of buffer time. If you've noticed the red flag at all, you've already won half the battle. Now you can make a note—here's where one of your rare, one-word reminders on a pad of paper is warranted—to come back to this subject right after you hear about the sister's illness. Or you could jump immediately to the questions about blackouts, and return to pick up the rest of the family history later, time permitting. Even if you literally have no time to follow up on a red flag, the fact that you notice and remember it is important in itself. You can still discuss with your examiners what additional information you might have learned had you had time to dig more deeply. Tell them how diagnosis and treatment could be affected by what you might have heard.

If the Patient Resists

Although most Board examination patients will cooperate throughout the interview, a few may offer resistance of one kind or another. A variety of precipitants can cause resistance to develop. Despite the fact that all have nominally volunteered, the occasional patient may have been under some pressure from fellow patients or treating psychiatrists. Another may have the flu or be experiencing side effects of medication.

Certain diagnoses make patients more likely to offer resistance. These include manic episodes, any acute psychosis, and antisocial and borderline personality disorders. Other patients may simply feel the need to conceal information—perhaps to make a good impression or to cover up shame. Of course, any of these motives may be compounded by how you react while taking the history. Without realizing it, you might express disapproval, either verbally or by gestures—frowns, shrugs, or any of the other idioms of body language we try to eradicate in residency, but that sometimes reappear during times of stress.

To counteract resistance, you first must recognize it. The clue may be as obvious as your patient's direct statement: "I don't want to talk about that" or "That makes me feel uncomfortable." But most patients don't like to defy doctors openly, so the message is usually more subtle: silence, a sudden change of affect, or body language of the patient's own such as downcast eyes or frequent glances at the examiners or at a wristwatch. A patient may also complain about missing lunch or a therapy session, or may ask to use the bathroom or to smoke a cigarette. Vague answers to questions or the inability to remember details that should be familiar are other means by which patients may tell you that they don't want to reveal themselves further. Muteness can be due to severe psychopathology such as depression or psychosis, but it may be simply a device used by the patient to control the interview—the ultimate in nonverbal communication! Some patients may indicate resistance by nothing more than a slight hesitation before answering. As in any clinical situation, you will have to be continually alert to the nuances of the interchange between you and your patient.

Of course, you'd like to avoid saying anything that would precipitate resistance. But some subjects that may cause it are among those most important to cover in a diagnostic interview. Foremost among them are sexual habits and attitudes, psychotic thinking, suicide attempts, substance abuse, and history of criminality.

You will have to deal with resistance right away: you don't have the luxury of putting off sensitive questions until a second interview. If time is unusually short or the topic is not critical, you might first attack the problem by trying to change the subject. You could say, "I see that's a hard question for you. Maybe we should just drop it for now. Instead, let me ask you. . . ."

For example, suppose you discover that your questions about work history have rekindled the painful feelings of failure your patient had a week earlier when someone else got a coveted promotion. Because you don't have time to explore those feelings in any depth, and because you already have collected enough symptoms to diagnose major depression, you may want to back off and approach the work history from another angle. Ask how long your patient has been employed, or what the job entails. If you continue to elicit only silence, tears, or complaints, then you had better change the subject completely.

Always reserve the right to return to the topic later. Sometimes, a second try will be successful when the patient is more accustomed to you and to the interview situation. Even if you get no further the second time, you will have demonstrated your interest and perseverance.

If the question is especially important, or if the patient seems to be reacting negatively to the whole interview, then you must meet the challenge head on. Although you should try hard to avoid confrontations, you may have to make an exception if the patient appears restless, uncooperative, or otherwise uncomfortable. When it becomes clear that you are not getting the information you need, you can switch gears and comment on the patient's affect. Mention that you have noticed the silence, the change of affect, the vagueness. Try: "I notice that you are suddenly silent. Can you tell me what's wrong?" or "You look sad. What are you thinking about?" Because you've been getting nothing, you'll lose nothing by this maneuver, and a change of pace might help the patient to feel less burdened and more cooperative. Even a brief exploration of the patient's feelings or thoughts should reveal some clues to the reason behind the resistance. In turn, this may guide you to a resolution of the impasse.

In general, this is no time to explore whether the patient knows the reason for resisting. This line of inquiry is likely to be fruitless, anyway, and the clock is ticking. However, if you find yourself faced with a major roadblock (e.g., the patient becomes angry, sarcastic, or mute or tries to leave the room), you have little choice but to delve further into feelings. Usually, angry outbursts or sarcasm will be due to underlying psychopathology. If so, your patient may not be easily calmed with a few soothing words. But your inquiry may reveal a precipitant (something you said, something about your appearance) that you can discuss together and, with luck, set to rest. Whatever you do, don't allow your own anxiety to prompt a response that is itself hostile or angry. You are, after all, being tested on your psychiatric skills.

Vagueness

Vague responses may be encountered in patients who are mentally retarded or psychotic or in patients who have Axis II pathology such as histrionic personality disorder. But such responses may simply be another form of resistance that most any patient might use from time to time. Approximate answers (Question: "How long have you been depressed?" Answer: "A long time.") should be followed up with specific questions that suggest the range of answers you expect: ("A few days? A few months?") In similar fashion, patients who respond "I don't know" should be offered some choices before moving on to another subject. Ordinarily, you want to avoid any time-consuming confrontations over what the patient knows or does not know, but if your interview develops into a pattern of vague responses you should explore the reasons behind this form of resistance. Otherwise, simply make a mental note of the discrepancy between what the patient ought to know and claims to know, and discuss it with the examiners later.

Vague or circumstantial ramblings very early in the interview should prompt you to cut short the patient's free speech time and begin your focused, short-answer questioning. If vagueness forces this strategy, follow Sutton's law and "go where the money is": start right in asking about symptoms that will allow you to identify the psychiatric disorders you are most likely to encounter. These won't be much different from what you would expect to find in any other population of psychiatric patients. Mood disorders and psychoses will be most strongly represented, followed by personality disorders, cognitive disorders, and substance abuse, though not necessarily in that order. You will use your time most efficiently if you first ask screening questions for depression and psychotic symptoms: "Have you felt depressed, sad, blue, down in the dumps? Have you ever had experiences such as hearing or seeing things others couldn't see or hear? Have you felt people were following you, spying on you, talking about you, or trying to harm you?"

Even patients who are not notably vague, but who only enjoy a good chat, may need help keeping their answers short. This situation is most likely to happen during the early phases of the interview, just after the free speech portion. If your patient starts to tell you more than you need to know, don't be afraid to interrupt. Try: "I think I understand about your appetite. But has your sleep changed any?" (Notice that by asking a yes or no question you imply that now you would like a short answer.) An especially chatty patient may require several such interruptions before understanding how much you value brevity. A nod and a smile with each short answer should help reinforce the message that you want answers that are the "soul of wit."

Last Words

It is traditional in many training programs to close demonstration interviews with an invitation to the patient. This is usually something along the lines of "I've asked you a lot questions—is there anything you would like to ask me?" But the Board exam is not a training interview, and this question is one of the customary courtesies you should avoid. To obtain the maximum amount of information from your patient, keep interviewing until the examiners tell you that the time is up, and then stop at once. Express your thanks and show the patient to the door.

Special Constraints on Time

How you parcel out your time can be affected by other factors. We'll touch on two of them here—age and intellectual capacity.

The Geriatric Patient

Patients in the geriatric age group often present the person conducting a psychiatric brief interview with an embarrassment of riches: too much data. Not only can older patients have virtually any of the Axis I and Axis II psychiatric diagnoses, but because they have lived longer than the average patient, they have more experiences—both good and bad—to talk about. Their psychiatric conditions are also more likely to be complicated by medical disorders.

Plan to allow more time for reviewing personal and social histories. You may need to inquire about some experiences that would be less germane to younger patients, such as meal and food preparation, economic resources, leisure activities, and problems with transportation.

By the age of retirement, life often becomes dominated by losses: loss of health, jobs, income, and status. Older patients have lost friends and family to death; their children have moved away or might ignore them. Loss of income and physical functioning often means moving into a retirement home (loss of home). There may be no telephone, leading to loss of contact; the patient may no longer drive (loss of mobility). These are all facts of life for the older patient that demand special sensitivity from the younger interviewer, who may as yet have had little personal experience with loss.

Infirmity, with its attendant loss of control, leads to embarrassment. This in turn could result in some resistance, particularly in the form of denial. You may have to break through denial by being very concrete. For example, if your older patient denies your suspicion there has been no loss of contact with family, you might ask, "When did you last see your son?"

This may also be one of the few times when you find it expedient to share something of yourself or to allow some discrete physical contact—your hand on an arm—to help your patient feel that you can truly empathize. Speak slowly and clearly, but not too loudly. As one septuagenarian retorted during an interview, "Don't shout! I'm depressed, not deaf!"

Cognitive Disorders

Some disorders present the opposite sort of problem for the interviewer: too few data. These include mental retardation and dementias and amnestic disorders of various etiologies. Cognitive disorders not only create a difficult problem of differential diagnosis, but also may make it harder to obtain the history. You will probably realize early that the patient has a form of cognitive disorder, so you will already know a major portion of the diagnosis. You can concentrate on digging out information pertinent to its etiology.

These patients often think and speak slowly. Sometimes, they also do not speak clearly, which can frustrate an interviewer intent on reaping a bountiful harvest of information in 30 minutes. Don't condescend, and try not to rush. You are better off with less information, as long as it's accurate, than with a lot of information that's not accurate. To check on whether you have been understood, you may have to ask the patient to repeat your question. You may learn a lot just by verbally taking the patient through a typical day's activity.

In the rare, extreme case, you may not get much historical information at all. Then, whatever information you obtain must come from the mental status examination. Be specific and concrete. Here is a case where you will want to do the complete mental status exam, as outlined in Chapter 7. Remember, too, that you should be wary when you interpret your mental status findings. A person with normal intelligence would understand a shorthand phrase such as "hearing voices" to mean "hearing voices when there is no one around to speak." But a mentally retarded person might interpret it as nothing more exotic than hearing a normal conversation or the television announcer.

Finally, if you emerge from the half hour with fewer data in hand than you would like, try not to feel discouraged. Remember that no clinician, including either examiner, is likely to do much better with this sort of patient.

Chapter 9 ————————————————

Case Formulation

As the door closes on your departing patient, one of the examiners should ask, "Would you like a couple of minutes to pull it all together?" You bet you would! Here is your opportunity to think about the interview and to prepare your verbal presentation of the patient. If your examiners forget to ask you this question, it is perfectly acceptable to request the extra time.

Your examiners want to learn how you think about patients. Specifically, they want to understand the process by which you join the history you obtained with the observations you made during the interview to create a framework that will support a differential diagnosis. In the oral examination, this process is at least as important as the final result. Individual examiners may disagree among themselves about the most likely diagnosis, but they will generally agree as to the clarity of the thinking you used to get there.

You will be expected to integrate all the information you have obtained, weighing all the clues and balancing every finding, even when they contradict the emerging diagnosis or point to some alternative disorder. Most important, you must show that your initial thinking is broad enough to encompass a variety of (reasonable) diagnoses and that you do not allow certain data (such as the patient telling you the diagnosis of record) to stampede you into early closure.

The mental process of diagnostic decision making has been studied for years (Gauron and Dickinson 1966). The least suitable process calls for the diagnostician to decide early and then defend that diagnosis against new evidence. Another flawed strategy is to follow every lead on its own without trying to integrate it into a larger picture. The ideal diagnostic process calls for the progressive integration of data into a presumptive diagnosis that can be challenged or confirmed as new information emerges.

The material you select for presentation will provide the foundation for your differential diagnosis and *most likely diagnosis*. These in turn will influence your recommended therapeutic approaches. While you are thinking over these matters, the contents of this chapter should flash before your eyes. As you can tell from the length of the chapter, there is a lot to consider.

Making Diagnostic Decisions

Diagnoses are used for many purposes. Among them are planning treatment, advising relatives, discharging from hospital, filling out insurance forms, and communicating with other health care professionals. The process you use to make a psychiatric diagnosis for the Boards won't be much different than it is for any of these other purposes, but you will have to defend your reasoning publicly.

For any of the above-mentioned purposes, making a diagnosis today is far more important than it was when the psychiatry Boards were first given more than 60 years ago. Diagnosis then was not particularly useful for treatment, because there were no effective somatic or drug therapies. Insurance rarely paid for mental health care. Patients were less likely to be discharged from hospitals. And diagnostic criteria of the era (e.g., Bleuler's Four A's) weren't of much use in predicting the course of psychiatric disorders.

Evaluating Diagnostic Data

Even in the brief psychiatric evaluation, you will obtain a vast store of information from history and direct observation. Most of it will be interesting, and much of it will be valuable. But some of it will be vital to your diagnostic efforts. When you sift through this welter of information, keep in mind several principles of data evaluation.

History is better than cross-sectional observation. More than clinicians sometimes realize, psychiatric diagnosis depends heavily on the longitudinal course of a patient's illness. For example, what can you deduce when a patient reports hearing voices? Is the diagnosis schizophrenia, a primary mood disorder, somatization disorder, antisocial personality disorder, cognitive disorder, alcohol withdrawal, or some type of substance abuse? Even if you learn that the hallucinations have *first-rank quality* (e.g., two or more voices speaking in complete sentences outside the head commenting on the patient's activities), all you can really conclude is that the patient seems psychotic.

To select a most likely diagnosis, you need more historical information.

How long have the voices been present? Have they ever cleared spontaneously, or only with medication? What is their relationship to the use of alcohol or street drugs? Has the patient had other major health problems? Have the hallucinations always been associated with prominent mood symptoms? Family history and legal history also can strongly influence this differential diagnosis.

Recent history is better than ancient history. This rule holds for two reasons. First, symptoms that are reported early in the course of an illness may be too general to reveal much. Consider an adolescent with symptoms of anxiety and withdrawal. Will these symptoms develop into an anxiety disorder, are they the prodrome of schizophrenia, or are they an early stage of a depression that will later change to full-blown mania? Will they simply disappear as time goes on, to be recalled later only as a period of adolescent turmoil? Only the subsequent history is likely to give you a valid answer.

Second, recent history may include new symptoms that allow a more specific diagnosis or suggest a change in treatment. An obvious example is the patient who has had several depressions. Early in the illness they may seem to be unipolar, but years later a mania may finally appear. More frequently encountered is the patient with nearly any psychiatric disorder who subsequently develops secondary alcoholism. Simply stated, recent history is more valuable because it embraces a greater span of time.

Collateral history is often better than the patient's own. After all, patients sometimes don't have enough perspective on their own illnesses. Some may lie; others may forget. Even the most alert and best intentioned of them may lack important information that families can provide—psychiatric illness in parents or grandparents, for example. If nothing else, the collateral history provides a useful verification of the patient's version. In the ideal initial evaluation you would obtain information from the patient and from informants. However, the Board examination is less than ideal, and you will have to do without information from relatives, friends, physicians, and hospital discharge summaries. But remember that this material should be there. When the opportunity arises during your case presentation, tell your examiners that if you were treating this patient, you would want to have this information and explain what use you would make of it.

Signs are better than symptoms. Signs are better because symptoms (what the patient tells you) are subject to two separate interpretations: yours and the patient's. On the other hand, the signs (what you observe) of illness are less likely to be manipulated by the patient, with or without conscious motivation. Hence, another major justification for the free speech period at the beginning of any psychiatric evaluation is that it allows you the chance to note discrepancies between a patient's signs and symptoms. Here is a typical example:

> Your patient's complaints of depression and suicidal ideas are delivered with drama, considerable smiling, and the suggestion of seductiveness. You mentally move personality disorder nearer to the top of your differential diagnosis.

Objective findings are better than subjective judgments. Closely related to the signs-versus-symptoms principle, the argument favoring objective findings is, if anything, a little stronger. It reminds you to be wary of making diagnostic decisions based on intuition. (This insistence on diagnosis rooted in objective criteria is one of the principal virtues of the DSM-IV approach.) For example, the diagnosis of schizophrenia based on DSM-IV criteria has considerable predictive value; the diagnosis based on the clinician's perception of "schizophrenic feel" has little predictive value.

Crisis-generated data are suspect. Irrespective of any other clinical conditions or patient variables, fear can affect anyone's behavior, yielding distorted observations, forgotten experiences, and embellished stories. Thus, the narrative of someone who has just been jilted by a lover may be colored by a crisis-generated reactive depression. Retrospective falsification of historical data may accompany other negative mood states, especially anxiety and anger. But similar distortions may also occur under the influence of positive feelings such as elation and love.

It could be argued that a crisis sometimes reveals valuable information in the form of feelings and behaviors that would not otherwise emerge. Unfortunately, the one-interview format offers no reference point from which to judge the effects of crisis conditions on your patient's moods, attitudes, and behaviors. Although there are no data to demonstrate this point, we suspect that when a crisis does generate useful information, this information usually takes the form of observable behavior.

Characterizing the Valid Psychiatric Diagnosis

Selecting a good diagnosis should be no different in psychiatry than in any other branch of medicine. Of course, the first and thorniest problem is to decide what constitutes a good diagnosis. The test of goodness for most systems of classification is the ability to make accurate predictions. In the classification of medical diagnoses, this predictive ability is called validity. There can be no better beginning for discussion than to list the Robins and Guze (1970) phases for establishing diagnostic validity. These phases are described in greater detail in Appendix F.

1. Clinical description
2. Follow-up study
3. Delimitation from other disorders
4. Family study
5. Laboratory studies

What was stated originally by Robins and Guze in 1970 remains true today: no major psychiatric disorder has fully met all of the above criteria. (Possible exceptions are certain disorders such as Down's syndrome that most psychiatrists seldom encounter.) Diagnostic validity is not even guaranteed by inclusion in DSM-IV, which incorporates some disorders that have been validated less well than others. Unfortunately, that volume does not make clear which are the better-studied diagnoses.

If your working diagnosis is one that has been validated more completely according to the Robins-Guze criteria, you can have confidence in the predictions you make from it. For example, if you diagnose recurrent depressive disorder, you could reliably inform the patient about the course of illness, response to treatment, likely duration of episode, risk of recurrence, and risk of similar illness in relatives. Using carefully researched diagnostic categories will also help you feel better equipped to discuss the case with your examiners.

DSM-IV lists over 300 diagnoses. Approximately one-quarter of these could be considered discrete diagnoses; the rest are closely related, such as the subcategories of schizophrenia. Of the 300+ diagnoses, fewer than 40 may be rooted in adequate scientific study and therefore have good predictive value. Realizing that we risk criticism both for what is included and for what is left out, we present in Table 9–1 our list of the most valid psychiatric diagnoses. We have listed them in descending order of the frequency with which they may be expected in a general psychiatric setting.

The Differential Diagnosis

The diagnostic process begins when you greet your patient. From the first handshake, you are making observations, asking questions, and drawing inferences that will eventually lead you to your working diagnosis. This process is not a simple one, nor is it easy to describe. The practicing clinician does not function like a decision tree, in which key questions cause the interviewer to branch successively until the correct diagnosis has been ruled in. Nor does the clinician become a computer, number-crunching a giant database that contains the entire history to determine where the preponderance of symptoms lies. Rather, psychiatric diagnostics as practiced by the experienced clinician consist of successive approximations that develop from one or more of several possible areas of concern.

Although you will usually identify them early, these areas of concern can show up at any time during the interview. They include those areas that form the basis for the DSM-IV decision trees:

- Psychosis
- Irrational anxiety
- Mood disorders (depression and euphoria)
- Excessive somatic concerns
- Suspicion of cognitive syndromes

Table 9–1. Most valid diagnoses, in descending order of frequency, expected in a general psychiatric population

---

Common
  Major depressive disorder, single episode
  Alcohol dependence
  Bipolar mood disorder
  Schizophrenia
  Major depressive disorder, recurrent
  Somatization disorder
  Borderline personality disorder

Less common
  Panic disorder, with or without agoraphobia
  Dementia
    Alzheimer's
    Multi-infarct
    AIDS

  Antisocial personality disorder

  Obsessive-compulsive disorder

  Mental retardation, if specific etiology
    Down's syndrome
    Phenylketonuria

  Anorexia nervosa

Rare
  Learning disorders
  Gender identity disorder
  Tourette's syndrome
  Autism
  Delusional disorder

Source. Based on Morrison and Muñoz (1979).

To those we would add:

- Substance abuse
- Chronic legal and other social and personality problems

Each area of concern comprises a group of disorders that could cause the problem under consideration. Once they have been explored and the diagnoses have been arranged in order, with the most likely diagnosis at the top, they are called collectively the differential diagnosis. In arranging the diagnoses on this list, the clinician considers several hierarchies of desirability, which we discuss in the next few pages.

Diagnostic Hierarchies

These diagnostic hierarchies are organized around the principle that there is value in assigning some order of priority to any list of presumptive diagnoses. The main benefit is utilitarian: it promotes effective treatment and avoids giving the patient a pejorative diagnosis. But aesthetics also plays a role (a smaller number of diagnoses is more pleasing and intellectually satisfying than a larger number). In any event, these hierarchies provide a rational basis for choosing the most likely diagnosis and runners-up.

Hierarchies can be organized around any of several principles.

The principle of parsimony. This principle holds that, everything else being equal, it is better to explain all of the known facts with a single diagnosis than with multiple diagnoses. This idea, basically Occam's razor rehoned, was implicit in the writings of Kraepelin and was made explicit by Karl Jaspers around the middle of the twentieth century. Here is an example of the parsimony principle in action: a patient with alcoholism, depression, and auditory hallucinations would be diagnosed as having alcoholism with hallucinosis and a secondary depression. Many DSM-IV criteria recognize this principle by stating exclusion criteria. For example, a diagnosis of schizophrenia is not allowed if you can't rule out mood disorder.

The principle of chronology. For years, the sequence in which a given patient develops two or more psychiatric disorders has proven to be a useful framework around which to organize the differential diagnosis. The most obvious application of this framework has been to the diagnosis of mood disorder. Based on symptoms alone, competent psychiatrists may disagree as to whether a patient's depression is endogenous or exogenous, but they may more readily agree that this depression began subsequent to the onset of another disorder—alcohol dependence, for example, or a personality disorder. Some would call such a depression a *secondary mood disorder*. A mood disorder that arises de novo, without a diagnosable antecedent, would be termed a *primary mood disorder*.

The advantages of using chronology as an aid to diagnosis are clear:

- It increases the grounds for agreement between diagnosticians.
- It uses operational criteria for dividing patients into naturalistic groups.
- Identification of these groups helps to promote rational treatment.

For example, consider Mr. Brinker, who drinks heavily and is depressed. If he has primary depression and drinks because of it, you might want to treat him with antidepressant medication. But if he has primary alcoholism and a secondary mood disorder, you would probably want to get him off alcohol and take a wait-and-see approach to his depression. The chronology of the relative onsets of his drinking and depression is the critical factor that allows you to choose the better course of treatment.

The principle of the "safe" diagnosis.   The concept of diagnostic safety means that the patient is exposed to the smallest degree of risk. Faulty or improper psychiatric diagnosis can yield various untoward results. They include

- *Inadequate treatment.* The patient receives treatment that is ineffective or dangerous or fails to receive treatment that would be effective, or both.
- *Inaccurate prognosis.* The patient, the family, and sometimes even the physician are misled by a prognosis that is either too gloomy or too optimistic. Planning suffers: the patient lacks a solid basis on which to decide about marriage, childbearing, job training, purchasing insurance, and the myriad other decisions that might depend on accurate diagnosis.
- *Worsening symptoms from lack of adequate treatment.* Suicidal or homicidal ideas and plans may develop where there were none before. Auditory hallucinations may become insistent, and delusions may become more convincing and frightening.
- *Perpetuation of error.* The final danger is that once the diagnostic error is made, it will be passed along from chart to chart and from one physician to another.

The safety hierarchy limits risk by placing at the top those disorders that are most likely to remit spontaneously and to respond favorably to treatment. In essence, this is the concept of first making the more conservative diagnosis—operationally defined for any given pair of diagnoses as the one you would prefer for your own relative.

The subjective nature of this definition makes it hard to give an ordinal ranking for many diagnoses in this hierarchy. But most psychiatrists would agree as to which disorders belong at the two extremes of this spectrum and which should be placed in the middle ground. The details of this hierarchy can be debated endlessly and probably will be. Our proposed safety hierarchy is given in Table 9–2. Of course, mental disorders due to general medical conditions are always considered safe in that they usually resolve once the underlying condition has been effectively treated.

The principle of percentages. Finally, common things occur commonly. When all other guideposts to a good working diagnosis are missing, take into account how often you expect to encounter the diagnoses you are considering. Remember the adage, "When you hear hoofbeats in the street, think of horses, not zebras." It should remind you not to go beyond the obvious if you don't have to.

When you use this final principle, consider the diagnostic makeup of the patient population. Almost every patient interviewed for the Board examinations will be currently under psychiatric care. This means that if you use the principle of percentages to help decide your differential diagnosis, you must have a rough idea of the frequency with which the diagnoses you are considering occur in psychiatric populations. This may differ substantially from the frequency of the same diagnoses in general (nonpatient) population surveys. The

Table 9–2. Hierarchy of conservative (safe) diagnoses

Most favorable (most treatable, best outcome)
  Any disorder due to a general medical condition
  Recurrent depression
  Bipolar I disorder

Middle ground
  Alcohol dependence
  Panic disorder
  Phobic disorder
  Obsessive-compulsive disorder
  Anorexia nervosa
  Substance dependence (nonalcohol)
  Borderline personality disorder

Least favorable
  Schizophrenia
  Antisocial personality disorder
  AIDS dementia
  Alzheimer's dementia

latter show a high prevalence of anxiety disorders, phobias, and panic disorders, among other diagnoses (Robins et al. 1984). Percentage-wise, these disorders occur much less often in outpatient populations and are especially uncommon among hospitalized patients.

Our experience with over 2,000 psychiatric patients is incorporated into Table 9–1. The relative frequencies suggested there may differ from those you encounter, depending on the type of facility that supplies the patients for your examination. You will have a better chance of drawing a patient with schizophrenia or bipolar mood disorder if you are being tested in a public facility such as a Veterans, state, or university hospital. (Be alert: patients in these facilities may also have a variety of substance abuse and personality disorders.) If, on the other hand, the patients have been recruited from an outpatient setting, especially from a private or fee-for-service public clinic, your chances of interviewing one with a unipolar mood disorder or anxiety disorder will be enhanced. Another example of the percentage principle in action: if your patient is male, his chances of having somatization disorder are much less than for a female patient.

Although we know of no reliable data on this point, anecdotes suggest that sometimes those in charge of procuring patients for the Boards choose patients who are "interesting." That is to say, they do not conform to the specific rules of diagnosis we have discussed. Whether "different" (and difficult) patients are chosen or, as in real life, occasionally just show up, the moral for you is the same: zebras may be uncommon, but they're not extinct. If one trots by, be prepared to identify it.

Using the Principles as Guidelines

Each of these principles is only a general approach to solving diagnostic problems. None of them applies in every clinical situation, and none should be followed slavishly. (If this were not the case, we'd be giving the Boards to computers!) We can formulate a general approach to help us choose the rules that can best arrange the elements of a differential diagnosis into a descending order of probability.

1. Look first for a general medical condition. Derived from the safety principle, the logic of this first step should be obvious.
2. Because of its wide applicability and considerable validity (which stems from the fact that it uses longitudinal data), *chronology* is often useful. One example (alcoholism with depression) has already been cited. Other examples come to mind, many of which involve differentiation of primary from secondary mood disorders.

One of the best and most frequently encountered examples of the chronology principle is the co-occurrence of depression and multiple somatic symptoms. In such a case, a good history will help you pinpoint the most likely diagnosis. If the depression came first, you're dealing with primary mood disorder until proven otherwise. If the somatic symptoms have lasted a lifetime and have only recently been complicated by depression, somatization disorder with a secondary depression is much more likely.

3. If neither of the above applies, use *safety*. In many diagnostic situations, neither of the above principles applies—there's no hint of a general medical condition and precious little chronology to guide you. So next you should turn to the safety principle. Although this principle uses less information about the individual patient, it has the solidly practical effect of directing therapy to the most treatable diagnosis with the best prognosis.

Perhaps the most frequently encountered example is the patient whose agitated psychosis could be either mania or schizophrenia. The principle of the safe diagnosis asks you to consider schizophrenia second—or, better, last—after all other more treatable diagnoses with better prognoses have been eliminated. For example:

> Your depressed patient also has features of borderline personality disorder. From the history, you cannot tell how long the borderline features have been present. Because primary mood disorder is the more treatable disorder with the better prognosis, you decide that it belongs at the top of your differential diagnosis.

4. *Percentages* is the fallback position. If none of the preceding principles helps you to choose, you might have to rely on percentages, as in the following example:

> Mr. Taylor says his depression and alcoholism began at about the same time. (He meets full diagnostic criteria for both alcohol dependence and major depressive disorder.) Following the principle of the safe diagnosis (Table 9–2 suggests that primary mood disorder is the more conservative diagnosis), you would like to prescribe an antidepressant. But you worry that if Mr. Taylor does have a primary alcohol problem, you will encourage him to depend on medication and to ignore his responsibility for going to Alcoholics Anonymous (AA). What should you do?
>
> Your doubts may be partly relieved when you remember that only about 5% of male alcoholics also have a primary mood disorder. You decide that your best bet is to recommend AA first, and watch the depression closely.

In practice, the percentages principle is probably used a great deal more than clinicians generally acknowledge, but you should be wary of citing it during the exam. The examiners will greatly prefer that your working diagnosis be based on all the information concerning your patient's own history. If you must resort to statistics, be sure to justify your reasoning. Explain that you would be unlikely to make a definitive diagnosis based solely on probabilities. And you should also consider the importance of following a patient such as Mr. Taylor carefully, with the intention of changing tactics if it became clear that the depression did not improve as he dried out.

5. If *parsimony* applies, use it. An example was given earlier.

Other Diagnostic Considerations

Unfortunately, not all of diagnostics can be reduced to formulas. To every rule there are exceptions that require judgment based on experience. And some patients will test the mettle of the best clinicians.

Diagnoses Easily Overlooked

Some diagnoses are important to remember but easy to overlook. When you are preparing your differential diagnosis, be sure to consider the following:

- *AIDS and AIDS-related complex (ARC).* Even if they are far down on your list, mention them if they seem at all likely. They're on everyone's mind.
- *Substance abuse.* Never forget this one, especially in teenagers, but even in older patients.
- *Tardive dyskinesia.* There is an excellent chance that at some point your patient will have received neuroleptics.
- *Schizophreniform psychosis.* This one is really a temporary diagnosis to be used when you aren't sure whether the patient's psychotic symptoms mean schizophrenia or something else. It is there so you won't have to saddle anyone with a pejorative diagnosis unless the criteria fully justify it.
- *Mild mental retardation and borderline intellectual functioning.* These often-ignored conditions could explain stiffness of affect, "hallucinations" that don't seem quite psychotic, or a chronic course without evidence of chronic psychosis.
- *No mental illness.* This is a rare one. But those in charge of patient procurement have been rumored to press clerical workers into service when too few patients

show up. The diagnosis of NMI is uncommon in a psychiatric practice, but nearly every practitioner occasionally encounters a patient who has no psychiatric illness. And remember the uproar caused by psychiatrists diagnosing psychosis too quickly in the pseudopatients of Rosenhan (1973).

- *Undiagnosed.* It may require some courage to call a patient "undiagnosed" on the Board examinations, but it's a great way to start off any differential diagnosis when you don't know exactly what's going on. "Psychiatrically ill, but undiagnosed" is the ultimate in conservative medicine. It tells the examiner that you know the dimensions of the problem well enough to avoid being stampeded into a diagnosis. You will first establish all the relevant information. Of course, you'd rather not say, "I have no idea what's wrong with Mrs. Fields." But you might express your hesitation with something on the order of this: "Until we get information from her family (old chart, previous doctor, the laboratory), I think Mrs. Fields should remain officially undiagnosed. We should first rule out hyperthyroidism with a secondary mood disorder, and although schizophrenia remains a distant possibility, she'll most likely turn out to have bipolar mood disorder, manic type."

Surviving Diagnostic Uncertainty

On a single interview, you should be able to make a solid, valid diagnosis about 80% of the time. But for the other one patient in five, whether you talk for 30 minutes or 3 hours, you probably won't be able to make a valid, definitive diagnosis. The most common reason is inadequate information. However, we don't mean to imply that in such a case the interview wasn't competent. Even the best interviewers may not get adequate information from a patient who is disorganized, psychotic, secretive, or forgetful.

Just the opposite problem—too much information—is a second cause for diagnostic uncertainty. This embarrassment of riches yields multiple, often contradictory diagnoses. It can happen when the patient

- Tries too hard to please the interviewer by responding positively to nearly every question
- Is frankly confused about the history
- Deliberately obfuscates
- Has somatization disorder or some other condition that is commonly mistaken for other psychiatric illness

But even when the patient thinks clearly and reports accurately, you still may have trouble making a definitive diagnosis if the history or presentation is atypical. Example: A patient who has a long history of psychosis shows more affect or insight than is typical of schizophrenia.

The usual clinical solution to diagnostic uncertainty is to seek outside information. That is clearly impossible for you under the circumstances, but your evaluation alone may yet enable you to select a most likely diagnosis. One or more of the following factors may help:

1. *Length of illness.* Everything else being equal, several years' duration of psychosis suggests schizophrenia. For that matter, the longer *any* symptoms last, the more likely they are to continue. "The best predictor of future behavior is past behavior."

2. *More symptoms.* Even if continuous signs of the disorder have not been present for 6 months, as DSM-IV requires for a diagnosis of schizophrenia, your case will be strengthened if the patient has had, say, auditory hallucinations, three sorts of delusions, a schizoid premorbid personality, and a family history positive for schizophrenia. In a similar time frame, auditory hallucinations alone would make a less convincing case.

3. *Presence of typical features.* If at age 18 years a patient has had classical gunbarrel blindness and glove anesthesia, you will probably suspect somatization disorder, even if the review of systems falls one or two symptoms short of the full number required for that diagnosis.

4. *Absence of atypical features.* Your diagnosis will be more secure if there are no symptoms that suggest other more serious (or more treatable) conditions. In the previous example, you would be more reluctant to diagnose somatization disorder in the face of first-rank symptoms of schizophrenia or if there were classic features of mania such as hyperactivity, rapid speech, and euphoria.

5. *Response to treatment.* Even when you have little information other than a prolonged history of psychosis, you may not be completely lost. If your patient reports that the symptoms (you still don't know what they were) abated during 3 years of lithium therapy, no one would fault you for putting bipolar mood disorder at the top of your differential diagnosis.

Diagnostic Dilemmas

In addition to the diagnostic problems already cited, the practicing psychiatrist often encounters several other dilemmas. These usually involve conflicting diagnostic principles, and they must be dealt with on a case-by-case basis. We will mention a few of them briefly.

Alcoholism with psychotic symptoms.   Diagnosis is usually a problem only if the history is unclear. The conservative approach would be first to diagnose alcohol-induced psychotic disorder, with hallucinations, but of course it is far more common to encounter schizophrenia with secondary alcoholism. If you don't have enough history to make a clear decision, simply state what you would do in practice. In this case, you would probably first rule out alcohol-induced psychotic disorder, although you may well end up treating with neuroleptics and diagnosing schizophrenia.

Panic disorder with mood disorder.   The old DSM-III criteria (American Psychiatric Association 1980) stated explicitly that panic disorder could not be "due to another mental disorder, such as major depression, somatization disorder, or schizophrenia." Many physicians complained that they could not correctly diagnose patients who had mixed depression and anxiety states. DSM-IV has resolved this problem by eliminating many of the exclusion criteria that were common in DSM-III. Now, depression and most other Axis I disorders (except specific cognitive disorders) can be associated with panic disorder, agoraphobia, obsessive-compulsive disorder, phobic disorder, and even generalized anxiety disorder, provided the symptoms are not present *only* during the course of the other Axis I disorder.

Somatization disorder with primary mood disorder.   This combination represents a diagnostic-therapeutic tangle. Whereas treatment is supposed to depend on diagnosis, sometimes we allow the diagnosis to rest on the results of treatment. When discussing diagnosis during the Boards, you'd rather not fall back on recommending a therapeutic trial. But primary mood disorder is the more conservative diagnosis—it is more readily treatable and carries the better prognosis—so a patient with somatization disorder who has not been treated for depression may require one (or more) trials on antidepressants. But you should remember that a favorable result does not necessarily mean that there has been a drug response: somatization disorder patients not uncommonly improve, at least for a time, with any therapeutic intervention.

Depression with borderline personality disorder.   As the principle of safe diagnosis suggests, always suspect Axis I pathology before Axis II pathology. This is because you generally can't do much about personality disorder—not quickly, at any rate. If the patient is depressed and you don't have history adequate to decide which came first, you'll generally be safer if you list the more treatable diagnosis first.

Two personality disorders in the same patient.   Not all personality disorders are created equal; some have been better validated than others. The criteria for some are based on careful studies, others are based on theory or intuition.

If you believe a patient qualifies for more than one personality disorder diagnosis, you can choose one of the following with somewhat more confidence:

- Antisocial
- Borderline
- Schizotypal
- Schizoid
- Obsessive-compulsive

Recommending Treatment

Psychiatric management requires attention to these potential interventions:

- Biological
- Psychological
- Social

This *biopsychosocial model* has become the framework underlying modern treatment formulation. At all costs, you should discuss each of its parts in the treatment plan of any patient you examine.

At one extreme is the schizophrenic patient who may have an exacerbation after stressful emotional interactions at home: here, you might want to recommend treatment methods from each of the three categories just mentioned. At the other extreme, a patient with antisocial personality disorder may respond only to social interventions. But, to repeat, you should initially consider that all patients could benefit from each of these three vitally important components.

Here are a few questions that might help you select an effective treatment.

Are There Controlled Studies of Treatment?

Whenever possible, choose as your preferred treatment one that has been proven effective by controlled studies. Of course, nearly all well-controlled studies are carried out on series of patients with uniform diagnoses that have been made according to well-considered and carefully applied criteria. If you have followed the steps recommended in this chapter for a valid diagnosis, you are already close to a defendable, preferred treatment.

Are There Treatments Suitable for This Patient?

Almost any patient will benefit from some kind of intervention. For some patients psychotherapy works, but it is slow and uncertain. This is especially true for patients with personality disorders (other than antisocial personality disorder, which is unlikely to respond to any treatment, no matter how leisurely). But even for the antisocial individual, you can always recommend the education of relatives about the consequences of the disorder.

Still other patients (we are gradually moving toward the top of the safety hierarchy) may respond well to any of several therapies, none of which is specific for their disorders. Alcohol dependence and anorexia nervosa are two such conditions.

Finally, for some disorders there is specific therapy that, if it is not curative, is so thoroughly palliative that not to use it would be virtually untenable. Bipolar mood disorder and recurrent depressive disorder are prime examples of this category.

How Urgent Is Treatment?

Urgency can be evaluated in a number of ways, but most psychiatrists would intervene immediately if a patient faced imminent death (by suicide or homicide), crime, marital breakup, job loss, or progressively irreversible symptoms (as in a cognitive disorder). A bit further down on the scale of urgency would be evidence that the disorder was becoming worse, though not necessarily yet catastrophic. This evidence might include

- Worsening symptoms
- Increasing numbers of symptoms
- Increasing social and personal problems resulting from symptoms

Of still less urgency are those disorders and situations that may be inconvenient but don't produce much distress or maladjustment. Examples include the milder depressions, adjustment disorders, and a wish to understand oneself better.

In the case of coexisting presenting problems or diagnoses, you would generally attack the more pressing disorder first. But you must also consider the overall clinical picture; that means you still must decide which diagnosis is primary and which is secondary. For example, most psychiatrists would move quickly to restrain a person with primary alcohol dependence who has a secondary suicidal depression, but they would not immediately begin treatment with antidepressants or electroconvulsive therapy.

How Expensive Is Treatment?

Expense means more than dollar cost. It also includes an evaluation of the unwanted effects of somatic treatment or psychotherapy. As in any other branch of medicine, the test is: do the desired effects of the treatment outweigh its unwanted effects?

How Sure Are You of the Diagnosis?

Expensive, long-term, or risky treatments are attractive only in proportion to the certainty of your diagnosis. For example, you might recommend a therapeutic trial of antidepressants for a patient with somatization disorder and depression, but you would probably withhold electroconvulsive therapy, at least until you had better evidence that this patient indeed had two "primary" diagnoses.

Are There Contraindications to Any Therapeutic Modality?

Of course, you will consider specific drug interactions and allergies, but don't forget about

- Relative contraindications to electroconvulsive therapy
- History of noncompliance with drug treatment
- Problems that might limit the use of psychotherapy (such as low capacity for insight and lack of adequate insurance coverage)

Have You Considered All Feasible Modalities of Treatment?

It is rare that a psychiatrist feels equally at home with all the available modalities of treatment. Most of us specialize in one way or another. For that reason, gaps in the therapeutic armamentarium will sometimes develop; because we don't use certain types of treatment, we tend to forget that they can be valuable. The Board examination is no place to suffer such a lapse of memory.

What Has Worked in the Past?

If your patient claims that phenelzine previously helped but tricyclics have never worked, you will probably want to stick with success.

Treating With Medication

Somatic therapies are a consideration in the treatment of most patients today. You should always mention them, even if only to indicate why you plan to avoid them. If you propose to use medication, you might be asked to discuss a number of considerations specific to the drug you choose:

1. What is its specificity for the disorder? Some drugs are more or less specific to the disorders for which they are prescribed: lithium and bipolar mood disorder are one obvious combination. Other drugs, such as SSRIs and the neuroleptics, are effective in a broader spectrum of conditions.
2. How familiar are you with the medication? You're safer discussing those you know well through personal use.
3. Do you expect to prescribe the medication for short-term use or as maintenance therapy?
4. What form of the drug (tablet, capsule, liquid, parenteral, depot) would you prescribe, and why?
5. How would you initiate treatment? Gradually, as with an antidepressant, or more rapidly, as with a neuroleptic?
6. What are the important side effects, including those common to its class (e.g., dry mouth for the tricyclic antidepressants) and those peculiar to individual drugs (nephrogenic diabetes insipidus for lithium)?
7. How will you manage important side effects? These will range from the common (extrapyramidal symptoms) to the less common (central cholinergic syndrome) to the rare (neuroleptic malignant syndrome).
8. Is there a family history of favorable response to your drug of choice? The patient may not know, but you can point out that it is a question that you could also ask an informant.
9. Are there patient-specific indicators that would make you especially cautious in initiating treatment? These might include advanced age, kidney or liver disease, history of drug sensitivity, and pregnancy.
10. Does the patient want to take medicine? Has there been a history of noncompliance that suggests you should consider a depot neuroleptic?
11. What is the likelihood of abuse of the medication? Included would be the abuse potential of the drug itself, as well as the patient's history of abusing other drugs and of drug-seeking behavior.
12. Does the patient have a history of accidental or intentional drug overdose?
13. Is the patient taking other prescribed medications that might augment or interfere with the drug you choose?

14. Would blood levels help you arrive at an optimum treatment? This question could apply not only to lithium and carbamazepine, but also to some antidepressants.
15. How often would you administer medication (divided doses versus once a day)? At what time of day? On a routine or an as-needed basis?
16. Can you recommend simplification of the present regimen by eliminating any of the patient's present drugs?
17. If you recommend a change from the patient's present drug regimen, will it be within the same class of drugs or to one of a different type? Should there be a washout period between drugs? Should the switch be gradual? Or is the patient simply not taking enough of the present medication?
18. What are the legal ramifications of your recommended drug regimen? Issues might be the patient's right to refuse treatment, informed consent, and the management of the incompetent patient.

Psychotherapy

Most patients respond to verbal interactions. The usual question in a treatment formulation is not whether psychotherapy will be used, but what kind will be used. Here are some of the factors you might consider:

1. Which of the patient's main problems would be the focus of therapy?
2. What is the goal of your treatment? The range might be from mere palliation of symptoms to a total restructuring of personality.
3. How available for therapy is the patient? Would regular activities such as work or school interfere?
4. What is the patient's capacity for insight? Personality characteristics and intelligence would be two of the factors to keep in mind.
5. To what extent can the patient afford therapy?
6. What is your own experience and expertise with the form of therapy you recommend? For example, would you refer the patient for behavior modification, or would you do it yourself as part of a comprehensive treatment plan?
7. How well motivated is the patient, and what was the success of any prior attempts at psychotherapy?
8. Would you feel capable of working effectively with this patient, or do you sense a personality conflict?
9. What would be the potential problems and pitfalls of treatment? For example, how would the therapist's absence be handled?

Social Approaches

Environmental interventions may be critical to speeding up improvement, increasing the chances for survival in the community, or ensuring compliance with other interventions. Social interventions may be especially important for many of the patients seen in the institutional settings where the Board examinations are held. Consider the following questions:

1. Are there family or friends available with whom to work? Are they interested in the patient, and have they been helpful in the past? These people could assist with transportation and reminders to take medicine, and they could call the physician if the patient does not comply with the therapeutic regimen. Be sure to consider the benefits (and possible drawbacks) of including the patient's family and friends as allies in the therapeutic process. While you are presenting the treatments you would recommend, keep in mind how you would describe them your patient's family or friends. Some examiners ask their candidates to explain the proposed treatment plan as if the patient and family were in the room.
2. Would the patient profit from vocational rehabilitation?
3. Is the patient optimally placed? Would another type of residence be more suitable?
4. What sort of legal maneuvers might be warranted, either currently or at some point in the future? Included would be involuntary commitments, conservatorships, and fiduciary arrangements, as well as assistance with wills, durable powers of attorney, restraining orders, and divorces.

For convenience, we list the various therapeutic modalities in Table 9–3. Be sure to consider some from each of the three principal approaches: your patient may be quite ill and could require a variety of therapeutic modalities.

Assessing Prognosis

At some point during the half hour after your patient interview, you will probably be asked, "What did you learn in the interview that allows you to predict how well this patient will do?" Recall the various areas that are defined by the term *prognosis:*

1. *Symptoms.* Will they be relieved completely or only partly?
2. *Course.* Will the patient recover completely? Will there be only a single episode, or do you expect remissions and exacerbations? Do you expect chronicity?

Table 9–3.   Outline of psychiatric treatment modalities

Biological
  Drugs
  Electroconvulsive therapy
  Light therapy
  Psychosurgery
Psychotherapy
  Individual
    Cognitive
    Insight oriented
    Analysis
    Short term
  Group
    Disease oriented (Alcoholics Anonymous, lithium clinics)
    General medication clinics
    Family therapy
    General support groups
  Behavioral
    Simple reassurance
    Systematic desensitization with reciprocal inhibition
    Mass practice
    Ward token economies
    Thought stopping
Social interventions
  Vocational rehabilitation
  Social skills training
  Education of family
  Placement for acute, intermediate, or chronic care
  Involuntary commitment
  Conservatorship

3. *Restitution.* Will there be complete recovery, or will there always be residual pathology?
4. *Treatment response.* Will it be slight? Moderate? Complete? How rapidly do you expect the patient to respond to the various sorts of treatment you propose?
5. *Time course.* How long will recovery take, and what will be the interval before another episode (if any)?
6. *Social sequelae.* Will the patient's level of functioning return to the premorbid level? How will the illness affect family life? Job performance? Independence? Will financial support be required? What about legal problems such as commitment, conservatorship, entering into contracts, driving a car, and voting?

7. *Heredity.* How likely is it that the illness could be passed on to the patient's children?

Several factors will contribute to your estimate of prognosis. Among them are the following:

1. *Axis I and Axis II diagnoses.* The Axis I diagnosis is usually more important for prognosis. But personality disorders can also assume considerable importance, especially if there is no diagnosable Axis I disorder or if the patient rejects or otherwise frustrates attempts at treatment. Be sure that you explain clearly which diagnosis you have in mind when you are discussing prognosis.
2. *Duration of illness.* If the patient has already been ill for years, the prognosis for a complete recovery (barring a therapeutic miracle) is probably poor. But if the history has been a series of exacerbations with complete remissions, you can feel reasonably confident as you predict another cycle.
3. *Previous response to treatment.* As a predictor, previous treatment response is only as good as the previous treatment. If the patient has mania and has never been treated with lithium, you can upgrade your prognostic optimism by an order of magnitude, at least.
4. *Compliance with treatment.* As already noted, the patient's amenability to treatment may be affected by both the Axis I and Axis II diagnoses.
5. *Availability of treatment for the primary disorder.* This factor has two parts. a) Have effective treatments been devised? b) Considering the patient's own finances and geographic location, are any of these treatments likely to be used?
6. *Available social supports.* These may include families of origin, spouses, children, friends, support groups, physicians, and religious organizations. Generally, prognosis is directly proportional to the number of bridges the patient has left unburned.
7. *Highest recent level of functioning.* Axis V, the Global Assessment of Functioning (GAF), reflects the current need for treatment or care (Table 9–4). But the highest level of functioning in the past year also has prognostic significance because that is the level to which patients usually return on recovering from an episode of illness.

Note that this scale has been revised from the DSM-III-R GAF scale published in 1987. The revision extends even to the numbering system, which now ranges from 100 (superior functioning in a wide range of activities) through 90 (absent or minimal symptoms) to 1 (recurrent violence or serious suicidal act). When you discuss level of functioning with your examiners, it is quite acceptable, perhaps even preferable, to use verbal descriptions (e.g., low, moderately high) rather than numbers. Many of us have trouble remembering numbers.

Table 9–4. Global Assessment of Functioning (GAF) Scale

Code

100 | Superior functioning in a wide range of activities, life's problems never seem to get out of hand, is sought out by others because of many positive qualities. No
91 | symptoms.

90 | Absent or minimal symptoms (e.g., mild anxiety before an exam), good functioning in all areas, interested and involved in a wide range of activities, socially effective, generally satisfied with life, no more than everyday problems or
81 | concerns (e.g., an occasional argument with family members).

80 | If symptoms are present, they are transient and expectable reactions to psychosocial stressors (e.g., difficulty concentrating after family arguments); no more than slight impairment in social, occupational, or school functioning (e.g.,
71 | temporarily falling behind in school work).

70 | Some mild symptoms (e.g., depressed mood and mild insomnia) OR some difficulty in social, occupational, or school functioning (e.g., occasional truancy or theft within the household), but generally functioning pretty well, has some
61 | meaningful interpersonal relationships.

60 | Moderate symptoms (e.g., flat affect and circumstantial speech, occasional panic attacks) OR moderate difficulty in social, occupational, or school functioning
51 | (e.g., few friends, conflicts with peers or co-workers).

50 | Serious symptoms (e.g., suicidal ideation, severe obsessional rituals, frequent shoplifting) OR any serious impairment in social, occupational, or school
41 | functioning (e.g., no friends, unable to keep a job).

40 | Some impairment in reality testing or communication (e.g., speech is at times illogical, obscure, or irrelevant) OR major impairment in several areas, such as work or school, family relations, judgment, thinking, or mood (e.g., depressed man avoids friends, neglects family, and is unable to work; child frequently beats
31 | up younger children, is defiant at home, and is failing at school).

30 | Behavior is considerably influenced by delusions or hallucinations OR serious impairment in communication or judgment (e.g., sometimes incoherent, acts grossly inappropriately, suicidal preoccupation) OR inability to function in
21 | almost all areas (e.g., stays in bed all day; no job, home, or friends).

20 | Some danger of hurting self or others (e.g., suicide attempts without clear expectation of death; frequently violent; manic excitement) OR occasionally fails to maintain minimal personal hygiene (e.g., smears feces) OR gross impairment
11 | in communication (e.g., largely incoherent or mute).

10 | Persistent danger of severely hurting self or others (e.g., recurrent violence) OR persistent inability to maintain personal hygiene OR serious suicidal act with
1 | clear expectation of death.

0 | Inadequate information.

Source. Reprinted from the American Psychiatric Association: *Diagnostic and Statistical Manual of Mental Disorders,* 4th Edition, Washington, DC, American Psychiatric Association, 1994. Used by permission.

Chapter 10 ─────────────────────

Presenting Your Ideas

During the first half hour, the examiners have observed how you obtain information and interact with the patient. In the remaining time, they will want to see what you can do with that information—how you interpret it and how you would act on it. Specifically, they will want answers to the following questions:

- How well do you understand the patient?
- How well can you organize the material?
- How thoroughly do you understand the pathology you have encountered?
- Can you deal effectively with the concepts involved?

This chapter should help you present what you know so that it will show to maximum advantage.

One of your examiners will begin with some variation of "Please tell us about your patient." The next few minutes should be easy. Just present your patient much the way you've done dozens of times as a resident, first describing history, mental status examination, and verbal and nonverbal behavior, and then stating your conclusions. Try to adhere to several principles that will help improve your presentation.

Be succinct. Consider this: If you were an examiner, would you want to sit through 20 minutes of history and mental status on a patient you had just spent half an hour with? Well, neither do these examiners. They have a job to do, and their agenda includes more than just listening. And even if you could spin out your narration long enough to occupy the entire half hour (anyone who has ever sat for the Boards has had that idea—trust us!), you'd be doomed to failure.

Long-winded presentations are invariably interrupted by questions, leaving some candidates with the frustrated feeling that they have omitted much that was relevant and included much that was not.

You should be able to present the history of a reasonably straightforward patient in about 5 minutes. You can allow another 2 or 3 minutes for a complicated history, but in no case should you try to spend more than 10 minutes on your case presentation: you'd be telling far more than anyone could possibly want to hear. Remember that your job is not to give the unabridged, three-volume, original biography with footnotes—make it the *Reader's Digest* condensed version, instead.

You need an outline.   The outline you use for presenting the patient is not quite the same as the one you used to take the history. The order you should follow is pretty much the same as for any written case presentation (see Table 10–1).

There are nearly as many ways to present a patient as there are presenters. Because it seems smoother and better connected, we prefer the way that begins with the first episode of the patient's current (or, if not current, then principal)

Table 10–1.   Outline for case presentation

Identifying data

Present illness

Past history
  Psychiatric
  Medical
  Review of systems

Family history

Personal and social history

Mental status evaluation

Most likely diagnosis

Differential diagnosis

Formulation:
  Predisposing factors (e.g., genetic)
  Psychosocial stressors (e.g., abuse as child)
  Stresses that precipitated present illness
  Characteristic defenses—adaptive style

Workup you propose

Treatment plan

Prognosis

psychiatric illness and, through the inclusion of positives and pertinent negatives, brings us rapidly up to the present. Thus:

> Mr. Arnold is a 38-year-old divorced machinist who was well until about 5 years ago, when he suffered his first episode of psychosis. He had suddenly begun to hear the voice of God telling him that he was the Redeemer. In response, he quit his job and shaved his head so that he could join a religious cult. But the Hare Krishnas thought he was strange and referred him to the local community mental health center. There he was hospitalized for about 3 weeks and treated with several unknown medications. Mr. Arnold says he recovered completely and returned to work a month later. He remained well until about 2 months ago, when he noticed increased lethargy and trouble concentrating at work. . . .

You would then proceed to outline the symptoms and social consequencesof the patient's current illness episode. Note that this approach disposes of the identifying data in half a sentence and melds present and past psychiatric symptoms so that, as for many patients, there is no need to recount the past psychiatric history separately.

Some psychiatric histories are so complicated that they cannot be presented as a unified whole. Then, you will have to select one strand of the story as a place to start. Usually, this starting place will be the apparent onset of the symptoms that constitute the primary diagnosis:

> Miss Bartlett is a single, 23-year-old clerk-typist. Although she has been a heavy drinker since high school, she has had no apparent symptoms of alcoholism. About 8 or 9 months ago, Miss Bartlett stopped drinking altogether when she noticed that her word processor was transmitting special messages to her from Bishop Desmond Tutu. . . .

After describing Miss Bartlett's delusions and other details of her present illness, you could return to describe more fully her earlier history of alcohol abuse.

Notice that in each of these examples the presenter refers to the patient by last name and title (Miss, Mr., Mrs., Ms. Bartlett) and not by the too-familiar first name only. Also note that the patient is consistently referred to by name and title, not by diagnostic classification. "This 23-year-old schizophrenic" connotes an aloofness from the patient as a unique personality. Keeping your distance in this manner may be appropriate in pathology, but not in psychiatry.

We realize that this may seem to fly in the face of advice to "treat the patient as a tool to pass your examination," advocated in some Board review courses and to an extent implied earlier in this book (see Chapter 5). Think for a few moments, however, and the contradiction will disappear. It is perfectly possible to do an interview for some nontherapeutic purpose, while treating the patient with respect and not as a mere case or subject. Furthermore, your examiners will expect you to have this attitude.

Presenting the Background

When you present the personal, social, and family histories, you'll do well to follow the KISS principle: Keep It Short and Simple. You can briefly relate the highlights of your patient's life: place of birth, number of siblings and sibship position, parents' occupations, years of school, military service, marriage(s), children, and occupation. Beyond those bare facts, anything of relevance to the patient's illness you will probably have already reported in the history of the present illness. A sentence is enough to report any major surgical or medical events. If the review of systems is important (as it would be in the diagnosis of somatization disorder), you already should have mentioned it. This might be a good spot to slip in anything you forgot to include in the history of the present illness, but be sure to limit yourself to positives and pertinent negatives.

If there is no family history of psychiatric disorder, say so and move on. A positive family history, on the other hand, requires some care and thought. What you are striving for is evidence that will support your most likely diagnosis or will at least help you formulate your differential diagnosis. To that end, you may have to interpret the family history information you obtained. Can you take a brother's drinking and ultimate suicide as evidence of a mood disorder? If you think so, say so, but state your reasons. If you think that grandma's chronic psychosis was schizophrenia, say so, but say why. Your examiners want to know not only what you are thinking, but also why you are thinking it. When you make a deduction, explain the steps in your reasoning and don't make logical leaps. (This rule applies pretty generally throughout the Board examination.)

Your Deductions

While trying to arrive at your most likely diagnosis and differential diagnosis, you may feel hampered by the lack of some items of information you would have in a conventional consultation. Examples might include the following:

- Physical examination
- Laboratory testing
- Records from previous admissions

- Interview with parents or friends to check on compliance with treatment
- Repeat interviews to compare affective states and assess the stability of the history
- Personal interview with another relative to verify the family history

If you think you need more information, qualify your diagnosis as tentative and state what you need to make it more definitive. Examiners may not ask you for this sort of information, so you should keep it in mind and volunteer it at the appropriate time. However, if you state a conclusion without supporting data, most examiners will ask for the data (what did you observe or learn in the interview) that support your idea.

Finally, although you may be interrupted before you get there, plan how you will state your formulation. In two or three sentences summarize the major factors that bear on your patient's illness. For example:

> "In summary, this is a 35-year-old woman with a family history that strongly suggests mood disorder. She was well until about 6 months ago, when her husband left her for another woman. At first, she became depressed and then increasingly hypomanic. Although she denies she is ill, she now seems to be experiencing a full-blown mania. But because she was admitted just recently, I would want a blood level to rule out an amphetamine psychosis. With proper management, her prognosis should be excellent."

You can then fill in the remaining four DSM-IV axes and be prepared to discuss treatment when asked.

The Workup

"How would you work up this patient?" This is a question that you can reasonably expect to hear during your 30 minutes, so you should be prepared for it. Of course, you'll want to keep in mind all of the various maneuvers you could use to evaluate your patient further—those we've listed above. But you will probably be asked to justify what you propose to do, so you had better keep in mind several factors that may temper your enthusiasm for a particular procedure.

1. *Prevalence of the disorder.* Although pancreatic carcinoma is associated with depression, it is rare enough that you won't want to order serum amylase levels on all your depressed patients. As we noted in Chapter 9 in "The Principle of Percentages," to some extent prevalence will be reflected in the order in which you arrange your differential diagnosis. This would justify

deferring some of the more esoteric tests until you rule out diagnoses that occur higher in the differential.

2. *Whether the procedure would facilitate treatment.* Dilated cerebral ventricles have been found in patients with schizophrenia, but so far the association has been largely of academic interest. You would not depend on this finding to make or confirm a diagnosis of schizophrenia, nor would you defer treatment until you had the results of computed axial tomography (a CAT scan) or magnetic resonance imaging (MRI).

3. *Complexity of the illness.* A patient with a clear history of recurrent depression that responds well to medication will generate little enthusiasm for the "million dollar workup." But if your list of differential diagnoses is long, especially if it is headed by "psychiatrically ill, but undiagnosed" or by anything atypical, then your patient may require a more extensive evaluation.

4. *Value of the test.* How likely is the test (or whatever information you seek) to discriminate between entries on your differential? For example, although the dexamethasone suppression test may discriminate between certain types of depression, there are too many false negatives and false positives to make it a useful screening test for depression in a general population. (This statistical principle, referred to as Bayesian analysis, is discussed in Eddy and Clanton 1982. A fuller treatment is contained in the excellent [and readable!] monograph by Galen and Gambino 1975.)

5. *Cost of the evaluation.* Although financial reality is almost always mentioned last, it deserves early consideration in any discussion of the medical workup. It is noteworthy that some procedures with the greatest potential for delivering vital information (e.g., interviewing collateral informants) cost the least. Other methods are so expensive that, unless the patient has several insurance policies or wealthy and indulgent relatives, their principal effect in marginal cases may be akin to shock therapy.

Getting Along With the Examiners

Like everyone else, examiners come in a variety of types. Some will wander far afield; yours may stick pretty close to questions prompted by your own patient interview. Some like to press candidates to the limits of their knowledge; yours may let you relax once they have ascertained your basic competence. We know of one examiner who always bases his next question on the candidate's previous answer; another may seem to specialize in questions that come from left field. Some examiners are austere, others are friendly. But they all have this in common: they want to see your best efforts. They know you are nervous; they will not trick you. They want you to pass.

Have a Plan

Because you cannot predict what types of examiner you will draw, you should have a plan of action that will carry you through practically any situation. In general terms, we recommend what works best for most candidates—just be yourself. By that we mean to talk openly about what you know and how you reach conclusions. If you are open, candid, and, insofar as the situation and your temperament will allow, cheerful and friendly, you will feel better and you will help your examiners feel comfortable with you and confident of your abilities. If you've neglected to ask something, admit it—it's better for you to point it out than to have it pointed out to you. If something surprises you, say so. For example: "Mr. Evan's ability to do serial 7s seemed out of keeping with how bad he said his concentration was."

If you don't understand a question, ask for clarification. And if you find yourself getting into unfamiliar territory, admit that, too. If you don't take the initiative by admitting your oversight, it will soon become apparent anyway.

Avoid Playing Games

This exam is no place for psychological warfare. After all, the examiners are not the enemy. (If they were, they'd have the advantage of position!) This lesson was learned the hard way by a candidate who used a "sign" to deduce that one examiner was a psychoanalyst. The sign was that the examiner was wearing a bow tie (no fooling!). Using this information, the candidate "tried to tell him what he wanted to hear" about analysis. What the examiner heard was clear evidence that the candidate was neither an analyst nor terribly clear about psychoanalytic terminology.

Similarly, attempts at roundsmanship may fall flat. It doesn't hurt to slip a journal article citation into the conversation, when it seems appropriate. But there is no point in bashing your examiners over the head with your erudition. That is a situation where even if you win, you lose. If you have special expertise in the area that you are discussing, you are better off soft-pedaling your own accomplishments and showing respect for other points of view.

If you think we are advising you to be humble, you are almost right. No examiner wants to see a candidate fawn and grovel like Uriah Heep, David Copperfield's nemesis, but no one much cares for a braggart, either. Try to strike a happy medium. If what you've published is germane to the subject at hand, go ahead and mention it, but don't use it as ammunition for a battle. Remember that you haven't come to win a debate, but to be approved.

Listen for cues as to the examiners' interests and take all their questions seriously—even if they sometimes seem a shade beside the point. Issues you haven't previously considered can crop up any time, so you need a plan for how to handle them. Even if a question seems off the wall, resolve to regard it seriously. If you need a little time while you mentally switch gears, ask to have the question repeated or say, "Let me think about that for a moment." Then try to answer as clearly, succinctly, and pleasantly as you can.

Using Diplomacy

Dealing with examiners sometimes means walking a fine line. What differentiates mindless agreement from diplomatic avoidance of an argument? What is a proper insistence on your own ideas, and what is a reckless defense of your principles? These questions are difficult to answer in the abstract except to say that, when in doubt, it is better to err on the side of moderation and tact. It is even possible to be right about the facts, yet make such a mess of the question-and-answer session that you fail the examination anyway. (We presented examples of this sort of problem in Chapter 1.)

By now, it should be clear how strongly we recommend that you avoid unnecessary arguments. But that doesn't mean you should fall all over yourself trying to seem agreeable, either. If you feel duty bound to disagree, use some of the time-honored phraseology for doing so politely. Here are two examples:

"That's a good point, but. . . ."

"I'd also look at it this way. . . ."

Try to avoid "Absolutely not," "Never," "I disagree," and "With all due respect" (which usually is interpreted to mean "With *no* respect"). If you can cite a study as the basis for your conclusion, then do so. If you have to fall back on your own experience with similar patients, your position will be weaker and you may need to soft-pedal a little with something on the order of "I've had some luck with carbamazepine in schizophreniform psychosis, but I agree that phenothiazines may be necessary."

Flexible Thinking

One of the more miserable feelings you can have as a candidate is to realize suddenly that you have been backing the wrong horse. In the context of the Board exams, that horse could be a diagnosis, a treatment regimen, or any point of psychiatric lore or science. To complete the analogy, your horse pulls up lame when a new thought occurs to you or when the examiner gives you some additional (possibly hypothetical) data.

Old adages to the contrary, this is exactly the point in your stream of thought where you should change horses. The examiner may be trying to test the flexibility of your thinking or your willingness to revise a diagnosis or treatment plan as new data appear. Here's what happened to one candidate who stubbornly stuck to one point of view:

> As related to us by the examiner, the patient was indeed depressed. But there were also a history of auditory hallucinations and a family history of chronic psychosis.

> CANDIDATE. The diagnosis is major depressive disorder.
> EXAMINER. Could it be anything else?
> CANDIDATE. No, just depression.
> EXAMINER. What about the voices?
> CANDIDATE. They're due to the severe depression.
> EXAMINER. What did you think about the family history?
> CANDIDATE. I thought there was psychosis due to depression.

> And so on, until the candidate ultimately failed the exam for want of sufficient flexibility.

If it is clear to your examiners that only one diagnosis is likely, you might safely keep your differential diagnosis list very short indeed. But your examiners want to be sure that you do not prematurely close the door on reasonable possibilities, so don't barricade yourself behind an untenable position. Instead, grab any chance to view your patient's problems from another perspective.

Some Don'ts and Do's

1. Don't throw terminology around. You won't win any points with psychiatrists by using psychiatric jargon, so save it for your next golf foursome. You are bound to lose ground with the examiners if you use terms you cannot define. So, if you feel tempted to say, "Mr. Lupus used the defense mechanism of projection," be sure that you not only can quote the dictionary definition of the term *projection* but that you also can cite an example from your own interview with Mr. Lupus.

2. Don't blame the patient. No matter how rugged the interview was, the patient is no longer present to mount a self-defense. Complaining will only detract from your professional image. This rule holds regardless of the circumstances. Even if the patient was tangential, even if the patient was mute, you only risk making things worse by casting blame. Besides, the examiners are clinicians themselves. Without any reminder from you, they know how

tough the interview was, and they will take it into consideration. So if you must, blame your therapist or blame your spouse (after the session, please). But don't blame the patient.

3. Do discuss the feelings your patient provokes in you, if asked. Counter-transference issues are fair game during the Boards. Your examiners may want to know whether you are tuned in to your own feelings about the patient, especially those that might make it difficult (or easy) to work with that patient in therapy. It is probable that to some degree you have already shown your feelings during the interview itself, so our advice is to adopt a policy of "measured honesty." We mean that you should own up to any feelings of uneasiness you may have, but that you should also temper your expression of these feelings with mercy. No one expects you to like a drug dealer or a rapist, but you won't gain points by showing undisguised contempt, either. "I might have difficulty working with someone with this pattern of charac-ter pathology" is an honest statement of doubt that no one could fault you for.

4. Do criticize your own interview. This guideline applies even if you think you did a splendid job. Even if the patient asks to see you for psychotherapy, *still* you should have the grace to point out some of your own deficiencies. A facility for self-criticism is an essential attribute for the complete physician, and your examiners know it.

5. Do mention material that you forgot to ask about during the interview it-self. This half hour is your second chance to cover material you might need to know about to make a diagnosis or recommend treatment, but didn't remember until the patient had left the room. Mention, for example, those parts of the mental status examination you didn't have time for.

6. Do respond to questions and to clinical issues as you would in practice. Candidates sometimes run into difficulty because they try to say what they think the examiner wants to hear. A recent example:

> Dr. Hogan works in a community mental health center, where he hardly ever orders psychological testing on his patients. Yet when asked whether he would do so for his Board examination patient, he replied, "Yes." (As he told us later, he thought it sounded right.) "Fine," responded the examiner, "Now, tell us how you would interpret the results." Dr. Hogan spent the next 5 (uncomfortable) minutes trying to justify ordering an expensive test he was not familiar enough with.

7. Don't ask the examiners how you're doing. They have been instructed not to say, and if they did say something, reassuring or not, it might give you false expectations.

8. Do cite medications and other treatments you use and are familiar with. You are more likely to be questioned on the treatment regimen you yourself have chosen.
9. Be able to discuss the laws in your state that pertain to psychiatric patients. These would include your duties to a patient, confidentiality, civil commitment, use of electroconvulsive therapy (ECT), duty to warn and protect (*Tarasoff* legislation), and issues pertaining to restraint and seclusion.

How to Respond When You Haven't a Clue

First, some preventive medicine: don't volunteer to explore uncharted waters. If you are not an analyst and you've avoided Anna Freud, you're better off staying away from the topic of the defense mechanisms. Remember that the examiners are there to look for areas of knowledge. Be sure you have some before you drop names or touch (however lightly) on any subject.

To be sure, you will often be unable to control the course of conversation, so you may find yourself discussing subjects on which you feel ill prepared. If in this sort of situation your first impulse is to wing it, swallow hard and reach quickly for your second impulse. Think about it this way. If you didn't broach the subject, then your examiners did. And they probably brought up the subject because they know (and care) something about it. With your certificate on the line, do you really want to fake it with a dedicated expert? There are better strategies.

When you are asked a tough question, remember that you don't have to answer immediately. It's okay to pause a moment for reflection. Don't worry about the pause—thinking before you speak is a positive attribute. If you like, you can fill some of the void with an honest "I'll have to think about that one."

Even a little information is better than none at all. If you have some idea as to a reasonable answer, mention what you know, prefaced by "I *think.* . . ." If you don't have the specific facts required but you can make a logical deduction, then do so, citing 1) what it is you lack, 2) the facts you have, and 3) the deduction. Thus:

"I've never used sertraline before, but I would guess its side effects are pretty much like those of the other selective serotonin reuptake inhibitors. So I'd warn the patient about nervousness and to be wary of insomnia, tremor, and gastrointestinal complaints—and to call me right away if any other problems develop."

Whether it is diagnostic criteria or a medication dose, if you are uncertain of the facts, emphasize that you would look it up.

Finally, keep in mind the twin principles that nobody knows everything and, in medicine, knowing what you don't know is vital. If the situation arises, you will find it far more satisfactory to demonstrate your understanding of these two principles to the examiners than to have the examiners point them out to you. If you are asked something you don't know, admit it, but explain how you would go about learning the answer if your patient depended on it.

Never fake knowledge you don't possess. Especially on the Boards, winging it is for the birds.

Chapter 11 ————————————————————

Surviving the Videotape Session

Videotaped interviews have been used to train psychiatrists for years, but for many candidates the first experience with an examination built around a recorded interview may come during Part II of the Boards. As a result, some candidates run aground on the shoals of this unfamiliar but basically straightforward examination format. With some instruction and a little cognitive rehearsal, you should be able to steer a safe course through the videotape examination.

Videotape Varieties

As you enter the viewing room with your fellow candidates, you should have several warnings clearly in mind.

This is not your living room. You could be distracted with noises from the air conditioner or from traffic outside. Someone may even decide to talk. And because the viewers will greatly outnumber the TV monitors, you may not be able to move to a better seat once the show has begun. So make a point of taking a seat from which you can see clearly and hear well. This will be especially important if you have impaired vision or hearing.

The show isn't Hollywood. In fact, it may not even be home movies: don't look for any fancy pans, lap dissolves, or fades to black. These tapes have been viewed by numerous psychiatrists, including your examiners (and, in some cases, by candidates of years ago). For the most part, the sound and image are clear, but you may occasionally encounter soundtrack static or a fuzzy picture. Try not to be distracted by the occasional technical glitch; concentrate on the material presented by the patient and interviewer.

You needn't expect Charles Grodin or Miranda Richardson in starring roles. No actors are used—only actual patients with real problems and real physicians with interviewing idiosyncrasies. As a result, you will see less than Emmy Award performances. This means that you may not get much in the way of affect and body language to help you with the diagnosis; it takes an actor to portray feelings in such a way that they don't flatten out when projected onto a screen. Most films do demonstrate important aspects of the patient's affect, although not all present a lot of identifiable psychopathology.

The interview itself may not have star quality.   You may find the interview unfocused, unstructured, and possibly uninteresting. Even examiners complain about the lack of information on some of these tapes. The one you see probably shouldn't serve as a model for your own live patient interview. If you were as vague and rambled as much as some video interviewers, you'd never get the information you need to pass the Boards. But the purpose of the interview is neither to teach interviewing technique nor to record the definitive exposition of a particular diagnosis, but rather to test your powers of observation and to serve as a springboard for discussion of general psychiatric issues. It will do that without fail.

Viewing the Videotape

Partly because most psychiatrists don't use it often in practice, the videotape creates anxieties all its own. In addition to the potential problems of picture and sound quality, you have no control over the interview. Lacking the flexibility inherent in interviewing a real patient, you must accept passively what is being laid before you. Then, you must try to process it, perhaps worrying all the while that the other candidates are somehow seeing more than you are. (They probably aren't.)

Furthermore, you may be denied the comfort of taking as many notes as you might like. In a darkened room with a videotape that cannot be stopped for an instant replay if you miss part of the action, you should feel reluctant to take your eyes off the screen even for an instant. Even if there isn't much activity, you don't want to miss anything. Although it seems unlikely that you would miss a clue that is vital to diagnosis, something important could get by you while you are scribbling furiously on a note pad. That's what happened to Dr. Macon, who related this story:

> From the direction my conversation with the examiners was taking, I knew something was wrong. They kept saying things like, "Did you see anything else on the tape?" Pretty soon it dawned on me that I hadn't seen quite enough! As soon as I figured out that I'd missed something, I said so. Then they told me what it was—the patient's father had died. So we discussed that for a while. I guess that in the long run it didn't make much difference—I passed—but that lapse of attention surely gave me some bad moments.

Other candidates have reported missing things such as tics that could indicate Tourette's disorder and gestures or facial expressions that suggested depression or other mood disorders. Although no candidate is expected to notice every single detail—the gestalt is what is most important—the more you see, the more complete that gestalt will be.

So our best advice is, don't take notes. Our second best advice is, if you must take notes, don't take many.[1] If you are afraid you'll forget some observation or idea, you can scrawl key words on a tablet. But don't try to write down everything. Limit your note taking to a single page. Don't worry about keeping it neat, and don't even think about looking away from the screen.

Organize What You See

So what's a candidate to do? How can you keep your eye on the ball yet remember every pitch, without taking the time to write it all down? Here's how we would go about it.

The organizing principle behind any initial psychiatric interview is your need to obtain two classes of information: the history and the mental status examination. We have already discussed their constituent elements in Chapters 6 and 7. You will be looking for the same information in a videotape interview. What's different—and in a sense much easier—about the videotape is that you don't have to think up your next question while you are trying to concentrate on the answers. Your only job is to organize and retain what you see and hear.

When you walk into the viewing room, have clearly in mind the various

---

1 Some examiners disagree. They feel that, unlike the live patient examination, candidates have more to gain than to lose from taking notes during the videotape. We agree that note taking is less dangerous during the videotape than during the patient interview, but we stand by our advice. You will have to make your own decision.

parts of the history and the mental status examination (see Table 11–1). As you watch the videotape, you will encounter bits and pieces of historical material that you will recognize as belonging to one of these subcategories. When you do, file them there—mentally—for use later. Of course, a relatively short interview like this one will leave a lot of gaps in the history. You may learn little of the personal and social history, perhaps nothing at all of the family history. There may be gaps in the present illness wide enough to park your car in. But after 20 minutes of even the most shapeless interview, you should know enough about the patient to present an outline of the present illness.

You'll probably get more from the mental status assessment. Work systematically through the outline, noting first what the patient is wearing and any peculiarities of behavior. Are there any abnormalities of speech? If so, jot them down in their appropriate place in your mental notebook. Next, pay attention to the quality, lability, and appropriateness of the patient's affect.

Content of thought may be a problem. Although the slice of interview you see may contain references to hallucinations, delusions, obsessions, phobias, or suicidal ideas, the topics of conversation are likely to be much more mundane, such as problems at work and problems at home. So when you do encounter definitive psychopathology, it is more important than ever that you note it for

Table 11–1. Outline for videotape viewing

Present illness	Mental status examination
Psychiatric history	Appearance and general behavior
Medical history	Affect
Review of systems	Type
Allergies	Lability
Medications	Appropriateness
Effects	Flow of thought
Side effects	Content of thought
Operations	Sensorium
Hospitalizations	Orientation
Major illnesses	Memory
Family history	Recent
Personal and social history	Remote
Childhood	Retention and recall
Occupation	Calculations
Military	General information
Legal	Abstractions
Marital and sexual	Insight and judgment
Personality, social, leisure	

future discussion. Here's the spot for the occasional one-word reminder on your notepad.

It is unlikely that the video interviewer will ask the patient to name U.S. presidents or subtract 7s, so watch carefully for any clues as to sensorium:

- Does the patient seem alert? Forgetful?
- Does the examiner have to repeat questions?
- Do discontinuities in the interview suggest that earlier material has been forgotten?
- Does the patient seem to comprehend everyday language, or must the examiner speak in unusually simple sentences to be understood?
- Are there references to current events or cultural material that help you understand something of the patient's fund of information?

Similarly, you may be able to infer something about insight and judgment:

- Does the patient seem to recognize that there is a problem?
- Was treatment sought voluntarily?
- Can you detect anything that would suggest compliance with recommendations for medication?

Using the Videotape Material

Just as would be the case during the live patient interview, you will probably be asked if you'd like a little time to organize your thinking. Most candidates want the time. Use the couple of minutes to review your mental notes and to organize your thoughts about differential diagnosis and workup. Then, you'll be as ready as possible to answer whatever questions come your way.

Your examiners will probably first request a general presentation of the videotape patient. Starting with the history of the present illness, work your way through the history (as much as you know of it) and the mental status examination. Be concise. There's a limit to the information you can wring out of a 20-minute, free-form interview, and you don't want to look like you're trying to pad the material. Work hard to include any major parts of the story (here's where your occasional, one-word, scribbled reminder might come in handy).

Do not overinterpret the data. If the patient talks about death, report just that, and don't infer suicidal ideas. If you think the patient was expressing covert thoughts of suicide, then say so, but preface it with "I think." That way, you'll avoid the implication that you can read minds. Some of the best candidates we have seen will volunteer what questions they would have asked to probe a point:

"If I had been conducting this interview, I would want to ask more about. . . ."

Keep in mind that an observation can have more than one explanation. The patient's motor restlessness could be due to anxiety, psychotic agitation, or akathisia from neuroleptic drugs. Without corroboration from the history, you'll be hard-pressed to choose the right cause. Play it safe and mention all that seem reasonable. The same holds true for diagnosis and differential diagnosis. But don't use a shotgun approach that includes every diagnosis imaginable: you want to show that you can evaluate information, not that you can memorize lists.

You may not have enough information to make a definitive diagnosis. If that's the case, you'd be ill-advised to choose one based on inadequately fulfilled criteria. When asked, list your complete differential diagnosis based on what you have learned. Be sure to volunteer why you hesitate to make a diagnosis and what questions you would like to ask (or diagnostic procedures you would order) to set your doubts at rest.

If you are asked to choose for further discussion one of the diagnoses in your differential, do as you are requested. Some candidates have come to grief because they feared they were being trapped, but your examiners have no such thought in mind. They only want some diagnosis (there's no such thing as the "right" choice) to serve as a vehicle for a discussion of issues such as workup, etiology, treatment, and prognosis. Any reasonable diagnosis could be the right choice, and the only wrong choice would be your refusal to choose anything at all.

Questions

Once you have come this far, anything is fair game. Here is a sampling of some of the questions you may be asked about the videotape:

- Did the interviewer and patient have good rapport?
- How might you have conducted the interview differently?
- If this were your patient, what would you do next, and why?
- How would you follow up on (any of the answers given by the patient)?
- Given only your present information, what would you do about treatment?
- Could you predict the course of psychotherapy for this patient?

We have presented the material specific to the videotape exam in a brief chapter, but we do not mean to imply that the videotape is not important to your evaluation for Board certification. Much of what we have said earlier—especially in Chapters 5, 9, and 10—also applies to the videotape exam. And of course, added to all the questions generated by the taped interview itself, you must be prepared to discuss the universe of general psychiatry, including its principles and practice, its science and art.

Chapter 12 —————————————————————

What If You Fail?

Now you've finished. Your two exam sessions are but fading memories. You've set your study notes aside to gather dust. All you have to do is sit back and wait for the envelope that announces your election as a Diplomat of the American Board of Psychiatry and Neurology.

Over the years that has been the experience of nearly 60% of the candidates who take Part II of the ABPN. (The actual numbers are given in Table A–1 in Appendix A.) But what if your envelope (they look just the same) contains other news? What does it mean? What are your prospects? What should you do?

To help answer these questions, let us first briefly review the overall evaluation process, which we discussed in detail in Chapter 4. After either session of the Part II examination (videotape or live patient interview), the two examiners who have been present throughout the session arrive at a consensus grade. If they cannot agree, the third (floater or senior) examiner acts as mediator until they do agree on a grade. This grade could be Pass, Fail, or Condition. The last is used for those candidates who are felt to be too marginal to pass, but whose performance on that segment of the exam is better than an outright Fail.

At a meeting of the directors that evening, the grades for the videotape and live patient exams are compared, and a final grade for the examination is derived. A Pass plus a Condition will usually, though not always, be recorded as an overall Pass. A Fail in either part or a Condition on both parts will result in a Fail for the overall examination.

As at any point of the credentialing process, candidates may also be disqualified for various sorts of unethical behavior. These include the following:

1. Presenting false credentials. For example, this might take the form of a forged certificate of residency training as evidence of qualification to take the Boards.

2. Possessing no unlimited license. This applies when it is learned that a candidate no longer has an unlimited license to practice medicine.
3. Cheating. The ABPN specifies the sort of irregular behavior that indicates cheating: copying, permitting another to copy from one's paper, and the possession of unauthorized copies of exam questions and/or answers. (Of course, none of these seems likely in an oral examination!)
4. Tape recording any portion of an exam session.
5. Attempting bribery.

The penalties for unethical behavior are severe, and the implications reach far beyond a single year's examination. Most of the above infractions will result in Board ineligibility for the next 4 years. In addition, the ABPN may send notification of its actions to the American Medical Association, state medical societies, and to other specialty societies.

Your Reactions to Failure

If you have recently failed the Boards, you can expect to feel terrible. That's the unanimous evaluation of all who have suffered this devastating experience. We cannot improve on the description of the emotional impact written by Lipp (1976), who collected questionnaires from 52 psychiatrists who had failed the ABPN on their first try.

> . . . It is apparent that being a Board Exam Casualty has a profound emotional impact on those who share the experience. All of the respondents experienced depression, some of considerable magnitude, although none reported suicidal ideation or abuse of alcohol or drugs. Overwhelmingly it was a lonely experience, to be shared openly with very few others. For many, shame, bitterness, anger, bewilderment, helplessness, and frustration were important themes that dominated their lives for months or years after learning their exam results. The personal and professional cost of these often painful emotional states is impossible to assess, but it would be fatuous to assume that the cost is negligible. Several casualties blamed their Board experience for major repercussions in their private life. Although the merits of any given case are certainly debatable, the painfulness of the experience for many can hardly be argued. (p. 281)

By the time he surveyed them, nearly half of Dr. Lipp's subjects had retaken the exam and become Board certified, but the bitter aftertaste lingered. Some noted that it had been the first failure of their professional careers. Others complained that certain career paths (such as teaching appointments) were now closed to them or that they were denied salary bonuses. Some blamed the ABPN itself for being controlled by psychiatrists "who are too far removed from real psychiatry" or for having a quota of candidates that it had to fail. (Neither of these accusations is true.)

From our own interviews with candidates, we know that Board failure can produce pain, depression, and shock.

> "I hadn't a clue I didn't pass." Dr. Williams fiddled nervously with her necklace as she related her experience. "There had been no conflict during the exam itself. I had a good patient and lots to say during the discussion. I thought 'til my head ached, but I couldn't see why they had flunked me."

(As we shall see, she learned the reason later.)

Many candidates develop significant psychopathology as a result of their experiences. Symptoms range from feelings of loss of personal or professional identity to varying degrees of depression to recurring dreams and anxiety states suggestive of posttraumatic stress disorder. Even those candidates who suffer least are affected to some extent:

> "I'm a good psychiatrist," one candidate told us. "I have a good practice, my colleagues respect me. But while preparing to take the Boards again, I had two recurrent dreams. In one, I was climbing a hill, naked. In the other, I was having to do gall bladder surgery!"

Where Do You Go From Here?

Even if you have not experienced the more glaring symptoms of some of your colleagues, you should still look for someone with whom you can discuss your feelings. We realize that it takes chutzpah to advise psychiatrists to seek psychotherapy—it's a bit like reminding a sanitation worker to wear rubber boots. But the published accounts we have read and the candidates we have interviewed have impressed us with the sense of isolation that develops among casualties of the Board examination process. You don't have to enter formal psychotherapy; just talking with a senior colleague may help you approach the certification process more realistically. So if you have failed the Boards, your first step to a happy resolution should be to find a sympathetic ear. Then, bend it—repeatedly, if necessary.

Writing for Information

When a patient's treatment isn't working out, the instinctive reaction of any physician is to ask, "Do I have all the information?" For a Board casualty, this translates to "What can the ABPN say that will help me understand why I failed?" Unhappily, the answer may be, "Not nearly enough." Here's why.

Over the years, the ABPN has tried telling candidates the specifics of why they did not pass. Some years ago that took the form of a narrative derived from the comments examiners had written during the exam. But as more information became available, it was increasingly disputed by candidates who felt they had been wronged. Board officials found that they spent more and more time, energy, and money defending their decisions. As a consequence, they now restrict the type and amount of information they release to candidates.

Many candidates would like the ABPN to return to its former policy of providing detailed feedback for those who failed the certification process. But most of the current directors of the Board appear to disagree. As Dr. Stephen Scheiber, the Executive Secretary of the Board, points out, "Other than its input into the standards for the training of residents, education is not a part of the ABPN mission." Some authorities fear that increasing the educational part of the Board's mission could distract it from its primary purpose and dilute its effectiveness as an evaluating body. Other specialty boards (for example, The American Board of Internal Medicine) share this assessment.

After a notice of failure is sent, a candidate has a month in which to request a performance evaluation. What can you expect for the $100 fee that must accompany your letter of request? You'll get a list of the six areas considered in the evaluation of every candidates performance. These are the same six areas that we have mentioned before:

- Physician-patient relationship
- Conduct of interview
- Observation of data
- Organization and presentation of data
- Phenomenology, diagnosis, and prognosis
- Etiologic, pathogenic, and therapeutic issues

On the form you receive from the ABPN, any or all of these areas may be checked as deficient on either your videotape or live patient examination, or both. But that's the only information you'll get. The Board of Directors continues to consider revision of its policy on feedback. But as of this writing, candidates who request an evaluation will receive no individualized comments, explanations, or suggestions for improvement. You will receive a letter that lists the sort of problems that candidates typically have with the exams. However, these comments will not be specific to you; rather, it is the type of information contained in this book.

You may ask, "Is this information worth the money?" It is a question many have asked, and one that we can't answer for you. If only one or two proficiency areas have been checked on your form, the information may help you pinpoint your difficulty and take corrective action. If most or all areas have been checked, the notice may leave you feeling little wiser than you were before. If you are the sort of person who feels uncomfortable passing up any possible shred of information, then you may want to gamble your $100 on the ABPN check sheet. But if you decide to do so, be sure to send your check right away. The clock for making that request starts ticking the day your notification of failure is typed. Your request for information must be received at the ABPN within 30 days from that date.

Should You Call the Examiners?

Absolutely not! In the past, some candidates have contacted examiners themselves (one of the Board casualties described in Lipp's paper reported doing so). However, several inherent disadvantages rule out this maneuver.

For one thing, there is the obvious demand on the examiner's time. More important for you is the time interval involved. After the examination, a month or more could pass before you would have cause to seek contact with the examiners, who by that time would have difficulty remembering in detail any one of the dozen or so candidates they had examined. Examiners do not retain copies of the evaluation cards they fill out, so any information they would be able to give you would be sketchy at best and possibly inaccurate.

Then, there is the question of how frank an examiner might be when confronted by an unsuccessful, possibly angry candidate looking for information. Although the Board examinations are by no means administered anonymously, their impartiality depends on the principle that examiner and candidate have no personal relationship. Like any other judge, an examiner is more likely to render an objective decision if there is no requirement to answer directly to the subject of that decision. Even if all these objections could be overcome, examiners (and directors of the ABPN) are admonished never to discuss the exam with former candidates. They can only advise you to contact the Board office.

The Mock Exam

You've probably already read Chapter 2 ("Preparing for the Boards"), so advising you to take a mock board exam may sound repetitive. But we can think of no other step more likely to give you the information you need. As an example, let's return to the case of Dr. Williams, whom we met earlier in this chapter:

In her previous preparations, Dr. Williams hadn't taken a mock board exam. Now, she sought out a senior psychiatrist who observed as she interviewed a patient. He had worked previously as a Board examiner, and he quickly pinpointed her problem.

"You've been interviewing too soft. You've sacrificed information for the sake of forming a relationship," he told her.

"And you know," she admitted later, "he was absolutely right. Thinking back on the patient interview I did for the Boards, I realized that I had been quite relaxed, and had behaved just as I would in my office. I spent far too much time trying to get the patient to like me. I gave up data I should have had, to get someone to like me whom I'll never see again. The patient was kind of vague herself, and I let her vagueness determine a vague interview."

With this lesson from her mock exam firmly in mind, Dr. Williams passed on her second try.

If you have already had a mock exam and you were told you passed with flying colors, we suggest that you take another—from a different examiner. Find one who's experienced and who will be tough. If necessary, call out of town to find someone you don't know. Because examiners are as human as anyone else, they will find it far more difficult to be suitably objective when criticizing the performance of a friend. More than ever, you want someone who can be totally candid about your interviewing skills and general psychiatric knowledge.

Your Best Response

With your mock board examination under your belt, you should then proceed as we outlined in Chapter 2. And you should begin preparing as soon as possible. After an experience as devastating as this one, your first impulse may be to put the whole thing behind you and not seek certification again. But the benefits of being a Board Diplomat are no less valuable now, only more difficult to attain. We recommend that you take steps immediately to "get back on the horse" before a phobia-induced paralysis of volition has a chance to set in.

The ABPN automatically schedules failing candidates for a reexamination. The date for this examination is usually enclosed with the notice of failure. It will be as soon as possible, but that is usually at least two exams—about 8 months—later. It will often not be in the same geographic region: ABPN gives preference to retesting candidates as soon as possible, rather than as close to home as possible.

Candidates are given about 6 weeks to tell ABPN that they wish to take the new exam and to pay for it (the reexamination fee is the same as that for the initial examination). Most candidates retake the exam. We strongly suggest that you send back the form, with your fee, right away, while your resolve is still high.

If the date slips by without action on your part, you will have to submit an entirely new application for Part II.

The success rate for candidates who retake Part II is understandably lower than that for first timers. Those who did succeed on subsequent exams reported that they were helped by several factors. These were evaluated in a survey of 339 ABPN Diplomats who had failed Part II at least once, but passed it subsequently (Table 12–1). No single factor dominated the list of reasons given, though most of the ultimately successful candidates thought that prior experience with the Boards was valuable. Note that feedback from the Boards, mentioned favorably by 38% of respondents, probably occurred during an era when more feedback information was given than has been the case recently.

Should You Appeal?

The ABPN has established an appeals process that is carefully thought out. It is also seldom used. Only about 1% of all failures leads to an appeal—perhaps six in the course of any given year. Although all sorts of problems with the exam process are alleged (e.g., "My grades must have been recorded incorrectly," "My patient wasn't any good"), most boil down to the candidate's statement that "I couldn't have failed—I left the exam feeling so good about my performance."

To appeal a failure, you must make a formal request through the Committee

Table 12–1. Reasons given by candidates for subsequent success after initially failing Part II

Reason	% of candidates
Having previously taken boards	81
Different examiners	66
Decreased anxiety	61
Additional study	59
Feedback from Boards	38
More appropriate patient	33
Additional clinical experience	31
Better exam environment	28
Additional colleague support	27
Board review course	25
Additional tutoring	24
Easier travel, hotel arrangements	11

Source. Adapted from Rudy and Kulieke (1981).

to Review Appeals, which requires that you submit your request within 55 days. If you decide to take this route, send your rebuttal information (the reasons that you believe should be considered) along with the fee, which is the same as that for reexamination: in the case of part II of the ABPN, it is currently $725. This committee will consider your evidence, rule on it, and send its recommendation to the full 16-member Board, which makes the final decision. That decision will be binding, both on the Board and on you. You will be notified by mail. (Although formerly candidates could appeal in person, with or without counsel, this practice was discontinued in 1988. Legal and stenographic fees were consuming too great a portion of the ABPN budget.)

As you consider this step, you should be aware that appeals are rarely successful. To be sustained, your appeal would have to present clear evidence that you were treated in a manner that was manifestly unfair. An example (to our knowledge never encountered) might be dismissal after only a few minutes of interview time. Examiners are so well coached during their indoctrination sessions that even minor procedural errors are unlikely. The chances of an impropriety severe enough to warrant reversal on appeal are vanishingly small. In fact, the staff at the ABPN could recall only a single successful appeal in the past 10 years.

Chapter 13 —————————————

A Mock Board Interview

This is a transcription of an entire mock board interview, conducted by a candidate who was preparing to take the oral examination the following month. The patient is a middle-aged white man, dressed casually, with no obvious mannerisms of dress, behavior, or speech. He had been well prepared for the experience by his own physician. We present the interview in its entirety, with only a few names of places and persons changed to ensure confidentiality. We also made occasional changes in grammar to promote easier reading. As the examiners make clear in their debriefing with the candidate, this interview was not especially well done, but neither was it a total failure. We chose it because we believe that there is a great deal to learn from the mistakes of others.

At the end of this chapter, we briefly discuss reactions of several anonymous Board examiners who reviewed this transcript before publication.

The Candidate Conducts the Mock Board Interview

CANDIDATE. Hello, I'm Dr. A.

PATIENT. Hi, I'm Mr. B.

CANDIDATE. And these two physicians will be observing. Did somebody explain the purpose of this interview to you?

PATIENT. *[Nods.]*

CANDIDATE. What's your understanding of that?

PATIENT. Well, I think you're going to take your credential kind of a test, and this is a process for you to get ready for your test and take the criteria you want

151

on this and you're going to ask me questions about my psychiatric history and try to get an in-depth view of what's been going on with me and—'cause you'll probably have to do this to somebody else to learn how to do it, and stuff.

CANDIDATE. Yeah, that's exactly right. Just so you understand that this is not a test for you in any way, this is a test for me for my certification in psychiatry.

PATIENT. Okay.

This is certainly the right gesture toward helping the patient feel comfortable. But has the candidate gone too far? This reassurance could have been given in a single sentence, with more time for gathering information.

CANDIDATE. Well, thanks for agreeing to participate. I'm going to be asking you a lot of questions over 30 minutes and we'll have to cover quite a bit of material, so I may need to interrupt you. That's just because we're very limited in the amount of time to cover a lot of area.

Smiling, the candidate does a good job of putting the patient at his ease and signaling time constraints and need for interruption.

PATIENT. Okay.

CANDIDATE. Okay, great. First, can I just ask you a little bit of basic information. Could you give me your age?

Is this a good beginning? A request for more general information about life and treatment problems would surely be far more productive.

PATIENT. My age—I'll be 33 this Saturday.

CANDIDATE. Okay. And are you working right now?

PATIENT. Yes, I am—part-time.

CANDIDATE. What is your job?

PATIENT. I deliver pizza.

CANDIDATE. Okay. And are you in treatment right now? In therapy?

Ignoring recommendations for opening with a period of free speech, this physician begins with four unrelated, short-answer questions.

PATIENT. Yes, I've been in therapy since 1978, but I've been in therapy with the VA since at least 1991.

CANDIDATE. Okay. And, uh, did you start therapy with the—

(To facilitate readability, we have deleted all subsequent use of "uh" and "ah," which were used with ever-greater frequency as the candidate became more and more anxious.)

PATIENT *[interrupts].*   Well, no, I've been ongoing for a long time, like in 1980 was my first thing with the VA. I was in the military from 1978 to 1979, and I was sick once before the military. My mother told me a lie—that's why I'm not getting benefits, just the hospital insurance.

CANDIDATE.   Okay, and you first started treatment in 1978?

The patient has volunteered this important statement: "My mother told me a lie." Will the candidate return to it?

PATIENT.   Right.

CANDIDATE.   Okay, what brought you into treatment?

Several minutes into the exam, here is this candidate's first open-ended question.

PATIENT.   Well, it's a long story. I was feeling a little bit depressed. If mother wanted to get rid of me, she put me in a mental institution. That was one of her ways of getting rid of me. I was a foster child. I didn't need the mental institution. All I needed was intensive outpatient therapy, because I'd never in my life committed suicide or been violent. But she just thought this is the best way she could get rid of me, and she was successful. I've never been the same since that hospitalization.

There is a great deal of feeling here, and the iceberg tip of a wealth of history about this patient's growing up. Does the candidate ever succeed in following up on this information?

CANDIDATE.   You were in your teens then?

The candidate has closed off the opportunity for more open-ended information and has missed the chance to develop more rapport with the patient with supportive statements such as, "You've been feeling bad for a long time" or "It must have been tough for you and your mother."

PATIENT.   Eighteen, yes.

CANDIDATE.   Eighteen years old. And what was going on with you and your Mom—going on at home?

PATIENT. Well, I was crying myself to sleep for about 2 years prior to that. I wouldn't talk to my parents about my problems because they wouldn't understand. I was dealing with everything myself. I wouldn't complain to nobody. I would just go home and cry myself to sleep. I was crying because I was very lonely, and then I had an episode of a crying fit on the telephone. That's when my mother brought me to—I only spoke to a social worker for about 5 to 10 minutes, and she had me put into a mental institution. I was also having a lot of problems at home, too, like my father. I saw my father looking at my sisters one day when they were taking showers, so I followed in the same footsteps.

CANDIDATE. What do you mean, you followed in the same footsteps?

Good use of the patient's own words to obtain details.

PATIENT. Well, I kinda hid in my sisters' closet, but I never saw anything. But I would do the same thing I saw my foster father doing.

The candidate never follows up on this revelation.

CANDIDATE. How long had you lived with that foster family?
PATIENT. Fourteen years.
CANDIDATE. Fourteen years. Okay. And when you're saying your mother, is that your foster mother you're talking about?
PATIENT. Right.
CANDIDATE. Okay. So you were feeling lonely and sad and crying at times at night. How long had you been feeling that way?

Good use of summary, to be sure that candidate and patient are talking about the same thing.

PATIENT. For about 3 years prior. I never tried to commit suicide. So I think that's a strong point for me. I'd never been violent or suicidal, so basically the psychologists don't really know what's wrong with me. But they give me medication and the medication I get right now is very helpful.
CANDIDATE. Good.

A more useful response: "How is the medication helpful?" (Does it reduce depression? Improve sleep?)

PATIENT. I go to school, also. I work part-time and I go to school, also.
CANDIDATE. All right. Let me just go back a little bit to talk about what was

going on at that time. So, for about 2 years you were feeling sad and you were put into a mental institution, you were saying? Where was that?

This patient has focused on presenting facts and avoiding feelings, so the candidate's use of a transition here is appropriate. But note the double question, with its potential for confusing the patient.

PATIENT.   That was in New York. It was called _____.

CANDIDATE.   Okay. And how long were you there?

PATIENT.   I'd say between 2 to 4 months. They had me drugged up—I really did know—I don't remember anything—and then I went to a private hospital for about 4 months. They gave me shock treatments at the private hospital.

CANDIDATE.   Okay. During—before you went into that institution, when you were living at home for those 2 years, were you having any other problems at home?

PATIENT.   Well, school was kinda hard. Like, my freshman year in high school I failed four out of five subjects, so the gym teacher kind of befriended me and we'd have something like therapy for awhile. The next semester I passed five out of five, and I only failed one the whole year. And what he was doing was trying to make my transition from junior high to high school a little easier. And I would cry to him. They were giving me psychological testing every year. I thought it was just to get out of class, but now I realize they knew something was wrong and they wanted to see what they could do to help me. But I think the psychological testing they were giving me didn't show anything because emotionally—I don't consider myself so-called mentally ill. I have a mental illness, but I'm not like most mentally ill people because I've always wanted to work. I've always wanted to go to school, and my stability has been on and off. That's why I haven't—I'm 33 years old, and I haven't succeeded much in a lot of areas. But the VA has helped me a lot. This is the first time I've been getting a shot. I've been getting a shot for about a year and a half. You see, the medication used to go through my digestive system and make me have physical side effects. I wouldn't take the medication because I didn't like the side effects. Now I get the shot and it just goes through my blood.

This is a terrific patient, knowledgeable, directable, and able to impart a great deal of information in a short period of time. In half an hour the candidate should be able to obtain virtually the entire history. The vast amount of information and its lack of organization will mean problems in presenting it, however.

CANDIDATE.   What shot is that?

PATIENT.   Haldol, 75 milligrams.

CANDIDATE.   Okay. And how often do you get that?

PATIENT.   Once a month.

CANDIDATE.   Okay. Well, it sounds like you've been motivated to do a lot for yourself.

The candidate uses this opportunity to say something complimentary and re-assuring.

PATIENT.   Always.

CANDIDATE.   At that time, when you were living at home, did you ever have an experience of hearing a voice or hearing your name called or—

PATIENT.   No. To this day I've never heard voices.

CANDIDATE.   Okay. All right. Did you have any other unusual experiences at that time?

Notice the manneristic use of "okay" and "all right," time-filling encouragements that are typical of an inexperienced interviewer who is trying to fill space while deciding what to ask next.

PATIENT.   Well, when I was in the military I thought I was the second coming of Jesus Christ and that I was going to be a rock-and-roll star.

CANDIDATE.   When were you in the military?

This virtual non sequitur leads the patient away from valuable information about psychosis the candidate has been trying to collect.

PATIENT.   From 1979 to 1980.

CANDIDATE.   Okay.

PATIENT.   I was 19 years old then.

CANDIDATE.   All right. Okay. And did they give you some treatment there?

PATIENT.   Yeah, they were trying all sorts of medication, and none of it was working. All they wanted to do was to make me stable so I could go to the VA in New York. I was in Virginia at the time. Then they moved me to—they took me to a place—I was on two plane rides, as a matter of fact. The first plane ride, there was nobody to pick me up, so they had to bring me back. And I stayed there for about 6 months, and the doctor took me off of everything completely. Two months later I was back in there.

When written down, many of this patient's speeches seem to show blocking. Neither the two examiners nor the patient's own physician felt that this was evidence of an actual thought disorder.

CANDIDATE. Okay. Now, I want to keep going back so I can get a little bit more information about that first episode when you were living at home. Did you have any periods where you weren't eating or you lost a lot of weight, or did you feel sad all the time?

Multiple questions again. Can we be sure the patient ever answered any of them?

PATIENT. No. I was wrongfully put in a mental institution, that's what it was. I didn't need it.

CANDIDATE. What do you think would have helped you?

Asking for an opinion when there is so much basic information to obtain is unwise.

PATIENT. Outpatient therapy. Having a concerned doctor, because the only question the social worker asked me when I went into the mental institution was, "Did I ever think of suicide?" And I told her I dreamed about it, and she put me in a mental institution. I think that was wrong.

CANDIDATE. Okay. But you've never made a suicide attempt?

PATIENT. Right. Not in my whole life. And also I believe going into the military was wrong, but my mother gave me the option: live on the street or go into the military. Even the military asked me three times before I got sick if I wanted out. I had no place to go, so I stayed in, and eventually I got sick. They didn't want to give me benefits, but they did give me hospital insurance, which is very helpful. I get to have good care, so it's very helpful.

CANDIDATE. Okay. I'm just going to ask you a few more questions about back then before we go back a little further, also. Did you have any periods where you would go for several days without needing to sleep or feeling very—

PATIENT. In the military I did. I must not have slept for 4 days straight.

CANDIDATE. Four days. Was that just one time?

PATIENT. Yeah, it was the only time I done that.

CANDIDATE. All right. And during that 4-day period were you doing anything unusual that you don't normally do?

PATIENT. I went outside with [just] my underwear on, one day. I cried for—I think I stayed in bed for those 4 days and I didn't eat anything.

CANDIDATE. And you were feeling sad during that time?

PATIENT. I think it was kind of a manic-depressive kind of a thing. I was going up and down—fluctuating. They also considered me a manic-depressive, but right now they have me diagnosed as schizoaffective. I think that a diagnosis where they don't know what's wrong with you. It's just a broad term, I think.

CANDIDATE.   Broad term. Yeah. It encompasses a lot of different kinds of problems. How do you see your problems?
PATIENT.   I'm schizoaffective, I think.

*To get the patient to explain how he sees himself was a good, but fruitless, effort.
Now the candidate properly moves ahead to gather diagnostic information.*

CANDIDATE.   Okay. Now, during that 4-day period, were you talking a lot more
than usual or doing a lot more things that you don't normally do?
PATIENT.   I was just crying a lot. My roommates didn't have a handle on me.
CANDIDATE.   Have you had other periods where you were very active or you
didn't sleep, or you felt happier than usual?
PATIENT.   I've never had symptoms like a manic-depressive. They sometimes call
me that, but I would never make a lot of phone calls. I would be like in a
manic state, a happy state, but I never got depressed where I would have to
commit suicide. I think I have a chemical imbalance in my brain. My doctor
tried to tell me in New York, there is a chemical called dorphormine [sic].
When I'm not on medication, it goes to my brain and makes me paranoid.
Somehow Haldol makes that able to control the dorphormine in my brain
so I can lead a so-called normal life.
CANDIDATE.   And you feel that Haldol helps you?
PATIENT.   Well, I've been on lithium and I've also been on Tegretol, but I'm not
on those right now.
CANDIDATE.   When were you on those medications?
PATIENT.   Tegretol. The VA in Omaha put me on that—that was I think October
of 1991—September to October of '91. They put me on Tegretol, and in
New York I was on lithium for a good 7 or 8 years, on and off.
CANDIDATE.   Were you on that alone or were you—
PATIENT.   It was Haldol.
CANDIDATE.   How did you do with—
PATIENT.   I stayed in the hospital for 5 years.

*The patient often interrupts, answering questions almost before they are asked.
This and the long, circuitous answers given at other times threaten to wrest control
of the interview from the examiner, who becomes visibly more anxious as the half
hour wears on.*

CANDIDATE.   Five years. And do you remember what kinds of problems you were
having while you were in the hospital?
PATIENT.   There were times I'd be too manic, like I'd be too hyper. I don't know
what the word means, but I would just feel real high.

CANDIDATE.   Real high?

PATIENT.   My main illness is paranoia. That's what brings me into the hospital—it's paranoia.

CANDIDATE.   Can you describe what you mean by paranoid?

This is a good attempt to check that the patient and candidate share the same definition of a crucial word.

PATIENT.   Well, I think cops are after me. I think people are talking about me. Now I think people are—especially the police—I feel when I'm around one they're looking at me for some reason, and to this day I really don't like police that much. But when I was in the military I was very paranoid, and I thought I was the second coming of Jesus Christ. I thought I was a rock-and-roll star. I didn't know how to deal with those, and the military didn't know how to deal with those, either.

CANDIDATE.   And this paranoia that you describe. Is that with you a little bit all the time or do you feel—

PATIENT.   It's a little bit with me all the time.

CANDIDATE.   And how is it affecting you right now, like today?

PATIENT.   Well, it's bearable. I take some medication, and it's bearable. Without the medication it excites me too much, and I can't stay in society. I have to go into the hospital. But if I see police I say, "Are they looking at me?" to myself. Where it gets—paranoia and depression is two serious words. Everybody feels down and everybody feels worried. That's where I'm at right now. I'm not paranoid, but I feel worried sometimes. That's the thing that I think that's normal.

CANDIDATE.   Right. Okay. And what do you get worried about?

PATIENT.   I just—I worry about people talking about me. I think my self-confidence is not that high. That's why I go through that. I think if I had self-confidence I'd do better.

CANDIDATE.   You feel your self-confidence is kinda low?

PATIENT.   Yeah.

CANDIDATE.   Why do you think that is?

PATIENT.   Well I really don't—I really don't like the way I look, that's one thing. I'm very shy around women, but not as much as I used to be. I've never had a girl friend. I've never been in a relationship. I have a woman therapist right now on the outside, not with the VA. We work on those things. I grew up being made fun of all my life, so when I went into some institution I—just being around messy old people and the way people treat you, you feel bad about yourself.

CANDIDATE.   What were you made fun of?

PATIENT. Well, my glasses, and I was called four eyes. My teeth were crooked, so they made fun of that. Things like that. Everybody had a nickname for me. If they wanted to laugh, they'd make a joke about me, and things like that. But it didn't bother me, and when I got sick, that's when it started to bother me. Normally I didn't care about how I looked—I thought I looked good. I thought, What the heck? At the mental institution I kinda started thinking about how bad I looked.

CANDIDATE. Okay, I'm going to interrupt you for a minute only because—

The candidate points out that a transition must be made, but neglects to make any sort of sympathetic comment on the obviously affect-laden material the patient has revealed.

PATIENT. I know I understand, you don't have to go over that.

CANDIDATE. Thank you. Now, have you had any periods where, for more than a week—let's say for many days or weeks, even though you felt sad almost all the time and you didn't feel good about yourself and you sort of felt like, what's the point of living? Have you ever had those feelings?

From the transcript, it is unclear which of several questions the candidate means to ask here. Although the patient seems to understand, a single sentence would have been simpler—and taken less time.

PATIENT. I've had those feelings.

CANDIDATE. And what's the longest that those feelings have gone on?

PATIENT. Probably no more than a week.

CANDIDATE. You never felt like that for more than a week?

PATIENT. Right.

CANDIDATE. Okay. And have you ever thought about hurting yourself? I know you said you haven't—

PATIENT. I have thought about it, yeah.

CANDIDATE. You thought about it. And have you ever thought about it over a pretty long period of time?

PATIENT. No, not for—about a week, at the most. Couple of days and it goes away.

CANDIDATE. It goes away? Okay. And what—have you ever come close to hurting yourself?

PATIENT. No. I don't like cutting my wrists; the only thing I thought about was taking an overdose of pills, but I never had any pills to take an overdose. I never had the possibility of doing it.

CANDIDATE. Have you thought about that frequently, or is it pretty rare that you think like that?

PATIENT. That's pretty rare.

CANDIDATE. Pretty rare. And what seems to make you feel that way?

PATIENT. My life—it's not worth living. Maybe I lost my job or I failed at school, or I'm very lonely and I don't see any girlfriend coming in the near future. I feel overwhelmed, and I don't want to get out of bed and I say to myself, "What's worth living?" and stuff. But I never came close to doing it.

CANDIDATE. Now, what you just described to me about how you were feeling— do you feel a little bit of that a lot of the time or is that—or do you not feel that way a lot of the time?

The long, double questions obviously don't confuse this patient, but they do take a lot of time to ask.

PATIENT. It's only a little bit that I feel that way. When days are going good, it doesn't even enter into my mind.

CANDIDATE. Okay. And right now would you say things are going pretty well?

PATIENT. Yeah. I'm going to school and working and stuff.

CANDIDATE. How long have you been at this job that you're doing?

A better follow-up on a new subject: "Tell me about your job."

PATIENT. About 3 months.

CANDIDATE. Three months?

PATIENT. Yeah.

CANDIDATE. And how is the job going?

PATIENT. It's going good. The place likes me, and I'm a good worker. This is going to be my first semester. It's ending this—next week. This is going to be the first semester I've ever finished in school.

CANDIDATE. Do these feelings that you described—feeling suspicious or worried sometimes—do those affect you on your job?

PATIENT. They are, but they don't affect me. I just deal with it like anybody else would.

CANDIDATE. Have you had other jobs before?

PATIENT. Yeah. I've had plenty.

CANDIDATE. Plenty. And what's the longest time you had?

PATIENT. A year.

CANDIDATE. A year. Okay. What job was that?

PATIENT. In New York I worked for a law school. I was in the graphics department. That was a good job, but social security wrote my boss a letter and everything went downhill from there. That was illegal, what they did, but they wanted to find out my job. And I was very fair with them and I told them, I didn't want them writing to my boss. But they wrote anyway.

CANDIDATE. And what led you to actually leave that job?

PATIENT. Well, I wasn't taking medication for 3 months, and I got sick.

CANDIDATE. Got sick means what?

PATIENT. I had to go into a hospital. I was getting paranoid.

CANDIDATE. Getting paranoid. Okay. All right. And what's the longest time you've been without being in the hospital?

This candidate continues to work too hard, thinking up question after closed-ended question. Better: "What was that like for you?"

PATIENT. Five years.

CANDIDATE. Five years. And when was that?

PATIENT. From 1982 to 1987, approximately.

CANDIDATE. Okay. And were you in outpatient treatment at that time?

PATIENT. Yeah.

CANDIDATE. Where was that?

PATIENT. New York. I was going to a clinic—I forgot the name of the clinic—and I was seeing a psychiatrist at the clinic, and he prescribed medication to me.

CANDIDATE. Okay. And do you remember what medications you were on at that time?

PATIENT. I was on Haldol and lithium.

CANDIDATE. Haldol and lithium. Okay. Right now you're only on the Haldol, is that right?

PATIENT. Right. And Haldol and Cognition.

CANDIDATE. Cogentin—okay. And the lithium was stopped when?

The candidate properly corrects the mispronunciation, to be sure that they both understand the same thing.

PATIENT. Lithium was stopped about 1989.

CANDIDATE. Okay. And do you remember why that was stopped?

PATIENT. I told my doctor I didn't want to take it and to take me off of it, and he did.

CANDIDATE. Okay. Do you know if you were having any problems with the lithium?

PATIENT. I was having—well, as I recall I was having—my enzymes in my liver were too high. That's why he took me off Tegretol.

CANDIDATE. Okay.

PATIENT. But the lithium, it was—I had to take 1500 milligrams a day for it to do good in my system, and that was too much. I was getting too many side effects like upset stomach, diarrhea, all that.

CANDIDATE.   Okay. And how have you done since the lithium was stopped?

PATIENT.   Fine.

CANDIDATE.   Fine. And have you been in the hospital since then?

PATIENT.   Well, I've been in the hospital in 1991.

CANDIDATE.   Okay, and what was that for?

PATIENT.   Paranoia.

CANDIDATE.   Okay. And you said you've never had the experience of hearing a voice or—

PATIENT.   Right. I think at Omaha they tried to tell me I did, but I really don't think so.

CANDIDATE.   Okay. Have you had any other, let's say unusual experience of thinking? That somebody else could hear your thoughts?

PATIENT.   I guess in 1991 I thought that.

CANDIDATE.   You did. Okay. And how about—did you ever feel that somebody else could put thoughts and ideas into your head?

PATIENT.   I thought that, too.

CANDIDATE.   Okay.

PATIENT.   I thought they were doing it by computer. By electrodes.

CANDIDATE.   Did you ever have the experience of feeling that somebody was controlling your body or your actions?

PATIENT.   No.

CANDIDATE.   Or your behavior in some way?

PATIENT.   No.

CANDIDATE.   Okay. Just controlling your mind?

PATIENT.   Right.

CANDIDATE.   And—okay. Have you ever felt that you were very powerful and you had some unusual powers that other people didn't have?

PATIENT.   No.

CANDIDATE.   You said you thought that at one time you were the Second Coming.

PATIENT.   I didn't think I had any powers; I thought I was just going to save the world.

CANDIDATE.   Oh. I see.

PATIENT.   I didn't think I had—like, I couldn't cure anybody or things like that. I just thought God picked me to be the savior of the world.

CANDIDATE.   Was that the only time that you had felt that way?

PATIENT.   Yeah. Well, see, it comes and goes, but it's never been to that extent.

CANDIDATE.   Okay.

PATIENT.   When I'm off medication, I get kind of rock-and-roll star. Not so much the second coming of Jesus Christ, but the rock-and-roll star comes into effect.

CANDIDATE.   What does that mean, the rock-and-roll star? You feel you are—

The candidate has a distressing tendency to ask a question, then try to answer it.

PATIENT.   Well, I'm gonna be on TV, I'm gonna be in front of people, I'm gonna sing. Stuff like that.

CANDIDATE.   Now, when you feel those ways did you ever—

PATIENT.   It's kinda manic, I think.

CANDIDATE.   Okay. Does that occur during a time when you're very active or when you're doing other projects than you normally do?

PATIENT.   It just happens when I'm off medication.

CANDIDATE.   When you're off medication. Right. And have you had periods where you've gotten involved in projects or a lot of activities that you don't normally do?

PATIENT.   No, not really. All I do is work and I try to go to school.

CANDIDATE.   Okay. Do you know if you've ever had periods where, let's say, you've spent a lot of money or made a lot of phone calls?

PATIENT.   No, nothing like that.

Patient has already stated this. But no one can be expected to remember everything from earlier in an interview.

CANDIDATE.   Okay, or traveled around to a lot of places?

PATIENT.   *[Shakes head.]*

CANDIDATE.   Do you think a lot about religion or a lot about God?

PATIENT.   I have a deep belief in God, but I really don't go to church every Sunday. But I do have a deep belief in God.

CANDIDATE.   Okay.

PATIENT.   And I—my morals and values are kinda connected with God. But I'm not a fanatic about religion. No.

CANDIDATE.   All right—

The patient goes right ahead, expanding on the earlier question. The candidate seems to be abandoning control of the interview.

PATIENT.   I don't like people who are fanatics about religion, and I don't like them to try and tell me about religion or about fanatics.

CANDIDATE.   Right.

PATIENT.   I've never been a Buddhist; I've never joined any cults or anything like that. I've been to different churches, and some churches I didn't like, so I left. And things like that.

CANDIDATE.   Okay.

PATIENT. I went to church every Sunday when I was a kid. With or without my parents telling me to go.

CANDIDATE. Is that right?

PATIENT. Yeah.

CANDIDATE. Okay. I'm afraid I'm going to have to skip to another area right now. I'd like to hear more, but there's a lot of information to go into, but we don't have very much time left. Okay. Let's see. How far did you go in school?

This speech makes the transition, but occupies far too much time doing so.

PATIENT. I'm in my first year of college right now.

CANDIDATE. Okay.

PATIENT. I graduated high school.

CANDIDATE. Great. Okay. And what are you studying right now?

PATIENT. Well, I'm just taking the basic courses right now, but just to let you know—I don't like talking about it too much—but I wouldn't mind doing something with psychology. Because I've been dealing with this for about 13–15 years, and I think I've learned something about it. That's what I want—

CANDIDATE. You've been through a lot.

The candidate interrupts for the first time in the interview, but makes an empathic comment that leads to more free speech, rather than using the opportunity to go for short answers that will answer diagnostic questions or cover other aspects of the patient's background.

PATIENT. Yeah. So, I think that I have enough intelligence. If I can get through school, I can do something with it. Lots of people have. Like, I've heard a lot of people who have gone through an illness and come back and written about it or taught it or worked in the field. That's what I want to do.

CANDIDATE. Great.

The manneristic responses "Great" and "Okay" continue to facilitate more speech without directing its content.

PATIENT. I don't know if it's possible, but I want to try. Because a lot of people in New York just tried to tell me it was impossible. And in California people tell me it is possible. So that's why I moved from New York to California, because I believe California has a different philosophy towards mental illness than New York does. New York is more institutionalized, then, and California's more therapy-oriented. I don't know if that's true, but this is how I feel.

CANDIDATE.   Okay. And you feel that you've been doing better since you've been here.

PATIENT.   Yeah. I have. The people that have supported me in California want me to succeed. I think the people in New York didn't want me to succeed because their egos were at hand and they didn't want to see me. Because at one time I was making more money than some people who worked where I lived, and the first chance they got they told me to quit the job.

CANDIDATE.   Okay. I'm sorry I'm going to have to interrupt you again. Now, do you recall why you were put on the long-acting Haldol—the shots? Were you having a little bit of difficulty taking your medication or remembering to take it?

Here is another long speech, culminating in a potentially confusing double question. Alternative question: "Why were you put on Haldol shots?"

PATIENT.   No, I was put on it because I was having physical side effects, and also the shot might be easier for me. I don't have to worry about taking it. But mostly because of the physical side effects.

CANDIDATE.   Okay. Were you making all your appointments—

PATIENT.   Yes.

CANDIDATE.   —and endeavoring to come, and remembering to come? And were you pretty much taking your medicine every day?

PATIENT.   I had a hard time with that.

CANDIDATE.   You did. Okay. Would you forget to take it or you just didn't think you needed it or—

With a great deal of information about medication already in hand, the candidate plunges ahead for more of the same.

PATIENT.   I'd probably forget to take it—more that I didn't think that I needed it. And then, there were times when there were too many physical side effects and I said, "The hell with it, I'm not taking it no more."

CANDIDATE.   Right, okay.

PATIENT.   But I always ended up in the hospital afterwards.

CANDIDATE.   Have you ever used any other drugs? Like street drugs?

PATIENT.   I smoked marijuana a little bit when I was 18, but that's about it. I never did cocaine or heroin or anything like that—

CANDIDATE.   Okay.

PATIENT.   —or pills. I never did anything like that.

CANDIDATE.   Drink any alcohol?

PATIENT.   I drank excessively when I was in the military, but I haven't got drunk since then. I drink a little bit. Like, I have, maybe one or two beers. But for

10 years I haven't gotten drunk or I haven't smoked marijuana. Things like that.

CANDIDATE. Okay. All right. I'm just going to ask you a few sort of standard questions, now. And just do the best you can, and I realize there is a lot of information about you that we don't have time to go over—

PATIENT. Right.

CANDIDATE. —but I just have to jump on them, because we only have a few more minutes.

The patient understands the need for speed, but the candidate plows right on with the full explanation. This would be appropriate for most interviews, but time here is of the essence. Alternative phrasing: "You've given me a lot of important information about your illness and background. Now I'd like to ask you some standard questions to see how clear your thinking is today."

PATIENT. Okay.

CANDIDATE. Can you tell me the date today?

PATIENT. *[Does so correctly.]*

CANDIDATE. Great. Okay, and what's the name of this place where we are?

PATIENT. *[States correctly the name of the facility.]*

CANDIDATE. Okay. And the state?

PATIENT. *[Gives it.]*

CANDIDATE. Okay. And I want you to repeat some numbers after me. Okay. I'm going to give you a series of numbers: one, nine, five, seven, three.

PATIENT. One, nine, five, seven, three.

CANDIDATE. Okay. Four, eight, two, six, one.

PATIENT. Four, two, eight, six, one.

CANDIDATE. Okay. Nine, three, one, seven.

PATIENT. Nine, three, two, one, seven.

CANDIDATE. Okay. Six, five, one, nine.

PATIENT. Six, five, one, nine.

One such set of numbers would easily have sufficed.

CANDIDATE. Okay good. Okay. Now can you spell *world*.

PATIENT. W-O-R-L-D.

CANDIDATE. And can you spell it backwards?

PATIENT. D-L-R-O-W.

CANDIDATE. Great. Okay. I'm going to give you four words to remember. And just repeat them to me first. Table, dog, rose, and carrot.

PATIENT. Table, dog, rose, and carrot.

CANDIDATE.   Okay. Let's try and remember them, and I'm going to ask you for them in just a few minutes, okay? Again: table, dog, rose, and carrot.

The candidate makes two mistakes here: asking for yet another practice repetition, and warning the patient that there will be a quiz later.

PATIENT.   Okay.

CANDIDATE.   Do you know who the president is right now?

PATIENT.   Clinton.

CANDIDATE.   Okay, great, and who was the president before Clinton?

PATIENT.   Bush.

CANDIDATE.   And do you remember who it was before that?

PATIENT.   Reagan.

CANDIDATE.   Okay, good. And do you recall what happened to Nixon?

PATIENT.   He got impeached.

CANDIDATE.   Okay, and what was the name of that whole—

PATIENT.   Watergate.

CANDIDATE.   Yeah. Okay. Great. All right. And I'm going to give you a little saying and maybe you could just tell me what you think it means: the tongue is the enemy of the neck.

PATIENT.   I would just say that some people talk too much.

CANDIDATE.   Okay. And, the grass is always greener on the other side of the fence.

PATIENT.   Everything looks better on the other side of the fence. Like, you're doing what you're doing, but if you'd like to be somebody else, it looks better. And so, that's what you would say.

CANDIDATE.   Okay, great. And if somebody said, "She's very level headed," what would that mean?

PATIENT.   She's very level headed. Very mellow—staying mellow.

Three proverbs would seem to be at least two too many. If further tests of abstraction are considered to be important, try asking similarities and differences.

CANDIDATE.   Uh-huh. Okay. Great. Did you ever have—when you were younger in terms of your schooling, you said you missed some grades or you failed some grades—did you ever get left back on any—

PATIENT.   No, not once.

CANDIDATE.   Okay. Were you ever in any kind of special classes?

PATIENT.   No.

This is an important area to cover, but it would have been better to learn about it before asking the mental status questions. To ask these questions afterward could imply that there was something wrong with the patient's answers.

CANDIDATE. Okay. And did you ever have a serious head injury?

PATIENT. No.

CANDIDATE. Okay. All right. Okay. Now, can you just repeat those four words back to me?

PATIENT. Table, chair, rose, and carrot.

CANDIDATE. Great. One of them was a type of animal.

PATIENT. Dog.

CANDIDATE. Great. Very good. Okay. All right. I guess we just have 1 more minute, so I'll ask you a few more questions. Tell me again how long you've been on the Haldol shot?

Still more questions about medication! There are a huge variety of alternative topics to tackle: What are your plans for the future? How is your relationship with your current therapist? How do you spend your free time? How do you feel about group treatment?

PATIENT. About a year and a half. Two years in October.

CANDIDATE. Okay. And how often do you go to treatment right now?

PATIENT. Well, at least once a month; maybe more. This month will be twice. I go to school, so I really have a hard time making it every week. But I definitely make it at least once a month for my shot.

CANDIDATE. And what do you do when you go to your treatment? What do you talk with your doctor about?

PATIENT. Well, I go to group therapy. I don't see my doctor every month. I just see one when I need to—

CANDIDATE. You go to group therapy?

PATIENT. Yeah. I have an individual therapist on the outside that I pay for.

CANDIDATE. Okay. Are you living by yourself now?

PATIENT. I live with two roommates.

CANDIDATE. Two roommates? Okay. And how long have you been there?

PATIENT. It's been a month—not even a month. I just moved in.

CANDIDATE. Okay. Well, thank you very much. Appreciate it.

PATIENT. Okay. No problem.

CANDIDATE. Nice to talk with you.

PATIENT. Okay.

END OF INTERVIEW WITH PATIENT

Examiners Interview the Candidate

The examiners offer a couple of minutes to organize thinking and notes. The candidate accepts.

EXAMINER 1.   You can start by giving us your summary of the case.

CANDIDATE.   Okay. Well, Mr. B is a 33-year-old white male who—unmarried white male who describes a long history of psychotic symptoms since about age 18. These include chronic paranoia with intermittent exacerbation into paranoid delusions. Other delusional symptoms including thought broadcasting and thought insertion and feelings of being mentally controlled, as well as grandiose delusions intermittently. He denies any history of auditory hallucinations and describes multiple psychiatric hospitalizations, some extending for several years, for what sounds like primarily psychotic symptoms with some affective symptoms. From his description—although I don't know completely how reliable the specific symptoms that he describes are—but from his description it sounds like he has not had a true episode of full-blown major depression or mania but has had intermittent depressive and possible hypomanic symptoms.

He has been on multiple psychiatric medications, including antipsychotics, Tegretol, and lithium. I don't have information on what happened with those trials or why he was taken off them—or exactly put on them—but he apparently had a problem with compliance in terms of taking his oral medication and was switched from oral Haldol to Haldol Decanoate about a year and a half ago. He's been in outpatient therapy off and on, and by his description he's been able to comply with that, although it sounds like right now he's primarily in group therapy rather than any kind of individual therapy. He goes once a month, and it sounds like he's very motivated to comply with his treatment at this point while he's on the medication at least. He has been doing well since he's been on Haldol Decanoate over the last year and a half.

He is currently living, in terms of his social history, with two roommates, but I guess he told me he's only been there for 1 month. I really didn't get information about his previous living situations or what happened with them. He said that he's never had a long-term relationship, and I think never been married, but I actually neglected to ask him about his social—other social contacts and friendships and other support system, including his family. He's had multiple jobs, it sounds like most of them short-lived and probably or possibly terminated because of increasing psychotic symptoms, although I'm inferring that from what he said, he didn't actually tell me that. He's had his current job for 3 months delivering pizzas, and he feels it's going well. He's in school, and it sounds like he's very motivated to continue with this and to keep functioning as well as he is.

He denies any history of recreational drug use other than a brief period of drinking while he was in the military in the late '70s in his late teens, and a little bit of marijuana usage around that time. I really didn't explore his family history or his early childhood history. Sounds like he was in one foster home and what preceded that—I don't have information about.

The examiners have allowed this candidate ample opportunity to present history freely. It is begun well enough with the history of the present illness and description of symptoms, including significant negatives. But as it progresses, a lack of organization becomes apparent. The candidate spontaneously admits to a number of omissions; this would have been more reassuring to the examiners had it been accompanied by a statement as to what use might have been made of the information.

Like Mr. B's speech, this candidate's own speech is somewhat rambling. The personal and social history is given in a disjointed way, again showing evidence of poor organization. At a minimum, it would have helped to announce the sections of the report as they came up: chief complaint, history of present illness, past medical history, personal and social history, and so forth.

EXAMINER 1. What would you have liked to have asked if you had time for that?

CANDIDATE. Well, I would have wanted to know if he was in multiple foster homes or in one, over a long period of time. What were his relationships with his family members? He said his mother put him into a mental institution against his will, and I would have wanted to know more about how that evolved and what his relationship was with that mother, and whether that was a long-term or short-term foster care, whether he had left previous foster care because of psychiatric symptoms, or whether there were other problems related to his home situation that I don't know about. And I would have wanted to explore why he was initially put into a foster home, if he had any previous history of—or his parents might have been psychotic or had other psychiatric problems, or other difficulties that made them not able to care for him. Whether there was any history of abuse that led to foster care or exactly what the reasons were and what the effect was on his—on his course. The other thing that I would have wanted to explore in that area would be more about his school and educational history. He struck me as, obviously, quite concrete, and I would just want to clarify—well, he denied that there was any past school problems or special classes or specific developmental problems related to that.

EXAMINER 2. What was concrete about him?

Here is a classic problem that candidates run into: the offhand comment that sounds good, but is difficult to sustain when challenged. With attempts at justification, this candidate becomes obviously more rattled throughout the next several minutes.

CANDIDATE.   Well, okay, let me—maybe I should rephrase that. His response— two of the three problems he responded to somewhat abstractly; only one he responded to concretely. But when I was questioning him, he—what appeared somewhat concrete to me was that he would give me multiple specific examples in response to a question rather than being able to sort of abstract the level of the question and answer it a little more succinctly.

EXAMINER 1.   Why don't you finish your past history and then go on to the mental status exam.

CANDIDATE.   Okay. Okay, the past history. Actually, I think that's all the past history that I have right now. With his multiple psychiatric hospitalizations, apparently some of them were for several years, including in a state hospital, and I would certainly want more information about all his hospitalizations and what kinds of symptoms he had and why he was hospitalized.

EXAMINER 1.   Would you like to report on your mental status exam?

CANDIDATE.   Okay. On mental status exam he was a well-groomed, pleasant, quite cooperative young man who appeared motivated for the interview. He had good eye contact. His psychomotor behavior appeared normal to me; it wasn't increased or decreased or any unusual gestures or mannerisms. His affect appeared slightly anxious but not dysphoric, and I'd say fairly cheerful and pleasant. His thought process appeared somewhat disorganized to me, in that he frequently sort of jumped around in the time frame, and in his response to questions he would not be able to really stay on track on terms of answering the questions specifically and in a succinct fashion.

The candidate has left out several important aspects of the formal mental status exam: appropriateness and lability of mood and flow of speech.

EXAMINER 1.   Do you recall an example of that happening during the interview?

CANDIDATE.   Well, when I asked him why he was in treatment now, he initially said that, I believe he said, that it was for depression—no, no, I'm sorry— when I asked him why he was in treatment he started talking about initially being in treatment in 1978 and then he was saying the military, and he was talking about his different hospitalizations, and about his mother and it seemed somewhat disjointed and a little bit disorganized or actually moderately disorganized, I would say, and—

To the examiners, the patient does not seem appreciably less succinct than the candidate.

EXAMINER 2. Can you say anything about his psychomotor activity?

The candidate had already covered part of this. The examiner is fishing for something else.

CANDIDATE. Okay. Well, his psychomotor activity appeared normal to me. Well, normal—he didn't have—he wasn't agitated. Possibly he might have been slightly on the decreased side. I didn't see any unusual mannerisms or gestures.

EXAMINER 2. What about speech?

CANDIDATE. Speech. His speech was clear, within normal rate and volume. He was fluent. It didn't appear pressured, and I didn't hear neologisms or paraphasic errors. And his thought content—he appeared not to have any delusions that I picked up during the interview. But he—at times when he started talking more about specific—what his job—I got a mild flavor of paranoid ideation. And that was subtle. I only noticed it once, and it occurred when he was talking about his jobs. He started to get a little bit pressured, and in his speech—and sounded a little suspicious, but there wasn't any overt delusional material.

The candidate never does mention the decreased latency of response, something noted by both of the examiners. Much of the mental status exam that did get done never gets reported: the examiners simply go on to other matters and ignore the sensorium. This can be frustrating to candidates, some of whom forget that their purpose should be to tell the examiners what they want to hear.

EXAMINER 1. Can you go on to formulate the case along psychological, social, and biological lines from what you know so far.

CANDIDATE. On terms of differential diagnosis I would say that he has long-term—

EXAMINER 1. Will you go on to formulate the case.

Examiner 1 restates the question to get the candidate back on track. There isn't a lot of empathy evident in the transcript, something about which many examinees complain. Examiners are instructed to be neither hostile nor overfriendly. Neutral affect is about as supportive as candidates can expect, under the circumstances.

CANDIDATE. Oh. Formulate the case. Okay. Well I'd say that this is a 33-year-old male with a long history of psychosis—of chronic psychosis—who had severe psychosis in the past leading to frequent hospitalizations and often extended hospitalizations. It sounds to me as if his functional level has been fairly low, although since he's been on the—on oral—on a depot neuroleptic over the past year and a half he has done better—quite a bit better—and has not been hospitalized over that period of time. He apparently has had problems with compliance over oral medications in the past which likely led to his—contributed to his—frequent hospitalizations and obviously probably led to the use of the Decanoate. He has been in outpatient and individual as well as group treatment and currently is in group treatment once a month in addition to his Decanoate medication and is probably doing well.

The candidate restates the present history, but does not volunteer important features of the formulation such as biological predisposition, psychosocial stressors, and defense mechanisms.

EXAMINER 1. Why don't we go on to differential diagnosis with him. Starting on Axis I.

CANDIDATE. Okay. Axis I. I would—the top of my differential would be chronic schizophrenia, paranoid type, and I would also want to get more information about his past history including all his records, and I would want to rule out a history of schizoaffective disorder. I don't—

EXAMINER 1. How would you go about doing that?

CANDIDATE. Well, I would want to know what the severity and also the length of his affective episodes were. He didn't describe any extended severe depressive or truly manic episodes in the course of his symptoms, but at times he gave some information which seemed—where he would say one thing which would be a little bit different from what he had said before. In terms of his course, I would just want to verify that with some past information—although in general I would say that he was a good historian and he was an able historian and he was able to remember his past—

Quite rattled by now (and this is only a mock board exam), the candidate rambles and repeatedly must be pulled back to the task.

EXAMINER 2. What else would you include in the differential?

CANDIDATE. Well, I would want to rule out—well, the differential would be delusional disorder; basically a chronic psychotic disorder with primarily paranoid delusions. I would include that because he denied a history of more bizarre delusions as well as auditory hallucinations, although it sounds like the extent to which his functioning has been impaired and also his behavior in general that it would really go beyond a delusional disorder into more of a schizophrenic disorder.

EXAMINER 2.   What else would you include in the differential?

CANDIDATE.   Well, I'd want to rule out bipolar disorder, given the fact that he does look fairly good right now. And I'd want to know if actually these psychotic episodes have occurred—he does describe here and there're a lot of affective symptoms. I'd want to know if they really primarily occurred in the context of prominent affective symptoms. So I'd want to rule out a bipolar disorder.

EXAMINER 2.   Did you get any information about that?

CANDIDATE.   About—?

EXAMINER 2.   Whether his delusions occurred in the context of affective symptoms?

CANDIDATE.   Well, I kind of attempted to get information about that, but what I did get was that he had periods of feeling sad and down and life was empty and that it wasn't worth living. And he felt lonely and isolated for long periods of time, but when I asked him about more vegetative—he even had some suicidal thoughts, although he says infrequently. But when I asked him about more vegetative symptoms of depression, he actually denied those. And he denied severe sadness or persistent sadness over extended periods of time, so it's really not clear to me how severe it was and what the time course was with those symptoms, so I'd really want to explore that more.

EXAMINER 1.   What do you make of his early history—age 16 to age 18? How does that fit into your differential diagnosis?

CANDIDATE.   Well, onset of paranoia, especially leading to hospitalization and I don't know what else actually contributed to hospitalization at the time, but that's the symptoms that he described that lead us to believe at that age would be more in keeping with chronic schizophrenic disorder. Actually, although it could still be consistent with the bipolar disorder or schizoaffective as well.

EXAMINER 1.   Any other diagnoses on Axis I? If not, you can move onto Axis II.

CANDIDATE.   I don't think there's any other that I can think of right now. Axis II . . . *[long pause].* I really don't—well, obviously he has this long history of paranoia. It sounds, with his hospitalizations and his level of functioning, it would go beyond a paranoid personality disorder and I really don't see anything else on Axis II that strikes me as prominent or—

EXAMINER 1.   Might you have you gotten any hints of traits or things?

CANDIDATE.   Well, he did talk a bit about his mother and his relationship to his mother—that she put him in a mental institution—that I really didn't explore. I didn't have a chance to explore his family relationships more. His reliance on people and how actually—what he uses for support at this time.

But I would want to consider dependent features of his personality, given his description of his relationship to his mother and sort of affective arousal when he was talking about it. He has been, I believe, fairly isolated, although that has bothered him a lot, so it appears that he does want more contact with people, so I'd want to consider avoidance features as well. Does he avoid social relationships because of a fear of being embarrassed or—there's a lot of social anxiety about relationships. And that certainly could be in keeping with his other problems.

The candidate's statement about not having the chance to explore the patient's background more is disingenuous: a great deal of time was spent unnecessarily on the medication history and portions of the mental status exam. It could be argued that there was probably much more drug history to obtain, but most examiners want to see that candidates know all the questions to ask, rather than witnessing an exhaustive review of any one area. Much of the candidate's discussion was regarded by these examiners as winging it. If you don't know, it's usually better to say, "I don't know."

EXAMINER 1.   Now let's suppose he's become your patient in the hospital. You're starting from where he is right now. Take your top Axis I diagnosis and tell us how you'd go about working him up. And then move on to how you would treat him.

CANDIDATE.   Okay. If he was in the hospital right now I think the top of my Axis I would be schizophrenia, chronic paranoid type, if he was in the hospital with acute exacerbation. And—but again I'd want to definitely rule out either schizoaffective or bipolar disorder as well as—I think I'd feel more sure that he goes beyond a delusional disorder. But I'd really want to explore the affective symptoms. What I would do is talk, first of all—get a better history in terms of his family relationships and other relationships, and try to get more information from any family members about his history. Collect his old records and also just explore with him in more detail about his affective symptoms in the past, see if I could get a better—

EXAMINER 1.   And what else would you do in your workup?

CANDIDATE.   Okay. Okay. Well, he—in his cognitive exam—well, one thing I would want to do is rule out any other causes for chronic or intermittent psychosis that would include, if he's never had it, probably a CAT scan and some blood work: B_{12}, folates, thyroid functions, and a basic chem panel as well as—

EXAMINER 1.   About the CAT scan—what sorts of things would you be looking for?

CANDIDATE.   Well, I think it'd be unlikely to show anything, given that he's had this for 18 to 15 years now. If there were anything treatable from a neurological point of view, it would have declared itself by now.

EXAMINER 1. And what might you be looking for?

CANDIDATE. What I would be looking for would be any evidence of—probably an MRI would be better—any evidence of past head trauma, of any, let's see—

In addition to a number of vague responses, the circumstantial, rambling way this candidate related to the examiners gave them the impression of someone who was not solidly informed about the matters being discussed.

EXAMINER 1. Any particular areas of the brain that might—?

CANDIDATE. Well frontal, temporal—changes suggesting some past injuries.

EXAMINER 1. Any particular side?

CANDIDATE. Oh. Well, I guess—I think it's left sided. Left-sided lesions are more likely to contribute to chronic schizophreniform type psychosis, so if he'd never had that I would want to get that. And then, there could be other— well I'd want to, for one thing, do a neurologic exam. Make sure he didn't have any focal symptoms that would suggest any specific lesion or organic for a long history of symptoms and nothing was declared itself as the first likely—

EXAMINER 1. How much are you going to do psychological testing with him?

CANDIDATE. Well, for one thing I think I'd want to get an IQ test to help assess what his potential would be in terms of vocational and that sort of functioning. How much might that contribute to his—any limitation in functioning that he would have. I know that sometimes it can be difficult to assess that without testing in a patient who has had psychotic symptoms, so that would be one thing that I'd want to do. I'd also want to, given his long history of psychosis, get some probably basic neuropsychological testing.

EXAMINER 1. What kind of tests would you be ordering and what would you be looking for?

CANDIDATE. Well, first I would want to do a detailed bedside screen of cognitive function, to see if anything looked abnormal or suspicious.

EXAMINER 1. Anything in particular; any particular tests you'd use for that?

CANDIDATE. That I would want to do?

EXAMINER 1. Uh-huh.

CANDIDATE. Well, I would want to do a basic detail cognitive exam, including probably more specific tests of attention, since he actually was borderline abnormal on the test of attention I gave him.

EXAMINER 1. Any specific test?

CANDIDATE. For attention?

EXAMINER 1. Uh-huh.

CANDIDATE. Well, I'd probably want to get him in a more relaxed environment and then repeat the digit span and then maybe do an A test on the basic screens of his attention.

EXAMINER 1. Okay. Now suppose your workup is finished, and you've decided that the diagnosis is chronic paranoid schizophrenia. What would you do as far as treatment?

CANDIDATE. Well . . . *[long pause]*.

EXAMINER 1. If you saw him as he is right now, what would you do?

CANDIDATE. Right, okay. Well, you know I'd first obviously want to collect all the information and be clear about what the diagnosis was and what his past response to various medication regimens have been and why particular medications were started and stopped; but, just based on the information I have now, it sounds like, with his very frequent and sometimes extended hospitalizations and his problems with compliance, I'd probably want to continue with the Decanoate medication and evaluate more extensively the affective component. If he's been doing well just on Decanoate for an extended period of time and he's functioning at a fairly good level for him and he feels pretty good, which it appeared he did today, then I really—and that's a stable pattern—then I wouldn't really see right now—

EXAMINER 1. What else might you do in addition to medication as far as treatment for him?

CANDIDATE. Well, what I would want to do is look at his environment and see if there's anything there which might contribute to intermittent exacerbations, anything that's stressful or unstable in his life situation— his living situation or relationships with family members or anything about his social or living environment that's chronically or intermittently very stressful.

EXAMINER 1. And what sort of treatment options might you offer him to assist with that?

CANDIDATE. Well, I'd want to get him connected with the social worker and somebody who could assist him if he needed any kind of help in terms of financial aspects or insurance, or, you know, that type of thing. And then I'd want to, you know, explore the possibility, if he needed it, of some kind of, you know, daytime structured situation or even more structured living situation.

Many examiners would like a more formal description of each proposed intervention, including identifying stressors or dealing with problems of interpersonal relationships.

EXAMINER 1. Such as?

CANDIDATE. Right now it sounds—although I have very limited information— he's only been living in this living situation for a month—I believe he said—

EXAMINER 1. Not the living situation, the other daytime structured environment you were mentioning. What were you thinking about?

CANDIDATE. Well, I was—I always want to consider the possibility of a day program or even not necessarily every day but maybe a few hours a day or a week to provide more social contact and feelings of being connected with people or a sense of belonging.

EXAMINER 2. Would you recommend any psychotherapeutic interventions?

CANDIDATE. I would, although again I—just based on the information I have now, I'd want to find out what's happening in his group treatment; why he's only in group treatment now. How he responded to that; how he was able to use that; has it been tried since he's been more stable—

EXAMINER 1. What kind of treatment would you offer him, and what would be the goal of treating him?

The questions might also be asked, "What were his feelings about his outside therapist? Group versus individual therapy?"

CANDIDATE. Well I believe that this basically—what I have now—that it would be primarily supportive. It'd be based on his problems in daily living and what kinds of things were stressful to him or, you know, on his mind or producing anxiety or dysphasia and things that bothered him. I'd try to focus on practical solutions for dealing with those. Maybe help him with some social skills that might decrease his sense of isolation.

EXAMINER 1. I'd like to know what your prognosis is at this point.

CANDIDATE. I think he's probably going to have continued intermittent and chronic paranoid symptoms now. Those—it appears to be minimized with the consistent use of medication and a good environment where there'd be more structure in his daily environment to help him maintain. I'm not sure yet, because I don't have those details, but I would say that he's likely to need some amount of structure and continued use of the Decanoate to maintain his highest level of functioning. And I would say, based on his past history, he'll have multiple hospitalizations.

It would be helpful to list signs, both positive and negative, that support the overall prognostic impressions. Also, what is meant by prognosis? Recovery? Ability to work? Social capabilities?

EXAMINER 1. I think we're about out of time.

CANDIDATE.   I'm just rambling on.

Insight!

                    END OF INTERVIEW WITH CANDIDATE

The candidate leaves the room while the examiners fill out their rating cards.

The Examiners Discuss the Candidate

After filling out their cards, the examiners discuss their rating of this candidate.

EXAMINER 1.   Oh man, that's tough. I don't think this was bad enough to fail, but—

EXAMINER 2.   I agree. I gave a pass on the physician-patient relationship with no problem. We saw good eye contact, and a lot of sympathy for the patient. Note taking was kept to a minimum, and wasn't intrusive. I think the patient felt pretty comfortable throughout. On the other hand, the interview initially was managed pretty well, but it got out of hand toward the end.

The examiner doesn't point out that, for the most part, this candidate also used language that the patient could understand and gave the impression of listening actively and attentively to the patient's story.

EXAMINER 1.   I thought it was a poor management of the time, because there was ample time to get a lot of the social history.

EXAMINER 2.   A lot of that got missed.

EXAMINER 1.   And there was too much focus on symptomatology and past treatment history.

EXAMINER 2.   I gave a high conditional there, because I did think that I saw the basic structure of the history.

EXAMINER 1.   Lots of people leave out at least one huge area. High conditional probably would go.

EXAMINER 2.   Family history was completely lacking.

EXAMINER 1.   Beyond knowing that he was in foster care. Military history also got left out. For anybody who a veteran, you should make at least some pass at combat history and PTSD, even though you don't think that's his diagnosis.

EXAMINER 2.   I gave a conditional on the organization of presentation.

EXAMINER 1.   Uh-huh. We had to spend too much time moving this candidate along from one section to the other. And the patient clearly said that for 2 years he was depressed and crying.

EXAMINER 2. But we also got the basic outline of most of the diagnoses that should be included in the differential, so I gave a pass on her diagnosis and prognosis.

EXAMINER 1. And I thought that we heard a reasonable treatment outline, and the biopsychosocial aspects were covered fairly well.

EXAMINER 2. I think that two other examiners could have failed this candidate.

EXAMINER 1. I think so. We've been quite lenient.

EXAMINER 2. Maybe too much so.

EXAMINER 1. I'm always being accused of being too lenient.

EXAMINER 2. Still, the way that I look at is that I think that this is a safe clinician, who was incredibly anxious, and, contrary to most candidates, whose anxiety level only increased as we went along.

Feedback Session With Candidate

EXAMINER 2. Tell us what you thought of your performance.

CANDIDATE. Well, I really didn't feel that good about it. I felt like I was disorganized and I couldn't do better. And I guess the other thing was that I felt like I should have explored more about his past.

EXAMINER 1. This should be a time for you to show how wonderful you are, not only as a diagnostician, but also as a clinician and as a person. Only a piece of this half hour has to do with data gathering and making a diagnosis. We want you to give us an entertaining and informative story about the individual who sits in this chair. We depend on you to formulate what's going on in the actual interview and present it in an interesting half hour.

Many examiners would disagree about "entertaining" and "interesting," but the balance of these statements would be generally agreed on.

EXAMINER 2. Keep us awake.

EXAMINER 1. Yes, keep us awake—keep us interested in you. That involves eye contact, use of voice, anything that it takes to make it come alive. Also, we want to know that you get a sense of who the patient is as a person beyond the illness and beyond the treatment.

CANDIDATE. Now, should you do that at the expense of getting diagnostic information?

EXAMINER 1. To some extent, yes. I think you covered all the big things about mood disorder and psychotic symptoms, and chronic hospitalization and medications, but I would have been much more interested in, say, his feeling about physicians that he worked with in the past. How did individual versus group therapy work for him? So that down the line you can at least get some indication of Axis II diagnosis. Also, sometimes when things are moving along, an examiner will ask you specifically what kind of countertransference issues you can visualize. Until you get a sense of how they interact with other clinicians or how you felt during the interview, you won't have a lot of data to substantiate what you might say about Axis II.

The examiner forgets to point out that the candidate also touched on the two major areas that must always be addressed: self-harm and substance abuse.

CANDIDATE.   Would it be okay to do the developmental during the time when you were going to do the history?

EXAMINER 1.   Sure. Anytime.

EXAMINER 2.   As long as you cover the material.

EXAMINER 1.   Yeah.

EXAMINER 2.   To drop the other shoe, the two of us would have passed you on this exam, but it was a close call, frankly.

CANDIDATE.   Oh, really?

EXAMINER 2.   And two other examiners, especially at the end of a long day, might not have been that generous.

CANDIDATE.   What can you tell me that's specific?

EXAMINER 2.   First of all, here's what you did very well. I thought you had good eye contact with the patient and you made him feel welcome. And you formed good rapport with the patient, I thought. Very clear pass on that. You had difficulty conducting the interview, towards the end especially, when there were still gobs of material that you needed. You let him talk too much. You should have kept right on going, down to the dot-dash, yes or no questions. Instead, you asked him four different sets of numbers, and I don't believe that we felt his cognition was that much an issue here. You did not get very much in the way of developmental data; you got nothing in the way of family history of psychiatric disorder.

EXAMINER 1.   Right. Especially for someone who is as articulate as he is. And if you've time left over, which is a common problem with some candidates, summarize his course of illness and current state in the last couple of minutes, saying, "Let me see if I've got this right." You should also remember to ask, "Is there anything important that I've left out that you think would be helpful?"

EXAMINER 2.   When you were presenting the history, you didn't give *us* much eye contact at all. You relied on looking at your notes. I think we both had the sense that your level of anxiety was increasing throughout the half hour rather than decreasing.

CANDIDATE. Really, yeah, I see this. Because I'm used to, most of my experience is hospital work, and I need to be collecting a lot of information around a problem and just, you know, really being able to organize it where I have all the information that—but I don't have time to organize it, I do get more nervous.

EXAMINER 1. I think that at one point you said that you would like to have gathered more data around—I forgot which particular issue it was—but it is helpful if you say, "I wasn't able to elicit this." And state what use would you have made of it.

EXAMINER 2. When it came to the discussion of MRI and other tests that you might do, I had the feeling that you were winging it. Now maybe you weren't; maybe you really knew where you were heading, but I didn't feel that you were confident of what you were saying.

EXAMINER 1. That was my concern. You might have said you were "looking for a left frontal lobe tumor because that's related to depressive symptoms." And we're going to ask you about psychological testing, even if you don't volunteer it. So be prepared to say, "I would order a memory scale because I was concerned about his memory deficit," or "I'd want an MMPI to see if he's at risk for suicide, because he seems to be presenting a very good face." So know what you're going to order and specifically what you're looking for. We have a problem with people who say, "I had the psychologist decide what sort of test to do."

EXAMINER 2. And then finally, on your recommendations for treatment, don't make us ask you about the psychological and the social. Sure, drug treatment is important, but the model is *bio—psycho—social,* so get it out there on the table. Then your examiners can sigh their relief and let you go early.

Wrong on one point: Examiners are cautioned never to let the candidate go early.

CANDIDATE. Now, are you really supposed to kind of present everything yourself, or should you wait until you're asked questions?

EXAMINER 1. We're happy if you can go straight through without our asking anything.

EXAMINER 2. Although we'll probably interrupt after awhile.

EXAMINER 1. I have a time frame for how long it should take me to present whichever piece I need. Five minutes for the history of present illness, another five putting in mental status exam and formulation, and so on. But I had the sense that you didn't have a mental image of the structure your interview would need to get through all the items of information. If you have any doubts about this, when you take your actual Boards, keep a list of the areas of the exam in front of you while you're interviewing. It'll help keep you on target.

EXAMINER 2.   Okay, any other questions?

CANDIDATE.   What do you think is the weakest thing?

EXAMINER 2.   From my perspective, there were two weak aspects. Of course, the formulation. But even more devastating was your control of the interview. Now this was a somewhat difficult patient; he had quite a push of speech, actually, which I don't think you mentioned by the way.

CANDIDATE.   Well, I thought he just talked like a New Yorker!

EXAMINER 2.   Well, actually, he had a decreased response time to questions. You'd ask a question and before you were finished it he was answering it. But that aside, you really didn't control the interview enough to get all the information that you needed.

EXAMINER 1.   And my biggest concern was that you didn't give us a feel for who he is beyond the diagnosis. You should not only know what the diagnosis, but what sort of a person he is.

EXAMINER 2.   My recommendation for you is this: dig up some more patients to practice on—maybe one every 3 or 4 days for the next several weeks. Spend half an hour just trying to get all of this information.

CANDIDATE.   Right. Can I just ask you two questions? How would you have interrupted him to structure the interview better, like what would you have said?

EXAMINER 2.   I would have said, "I'm sorry, but were really running low on time. Let me ask you a set of short questions." Then, as he gives you yes-no answers, nod your head or smile as you move right on to the next thing. By the way, you spent quite a bit of time saying, "Uh-huh" or "Yes" or "Okay." You were filling in with verbiage rather than having another question ready right then.

CANDIDATE.   In terms of your comments about knowing the patient better, what other areas do you think would have helped?

EXAMINER 1.   Who his friends are; how he spends his free time outside of delivering pizza and going to school; does he have friends in his classes; how did he feel at that time he said he had trouble in high school?

EXAMINER 2.   You're bound to get an examiner who wants to know all about this developmental material. What went on when he was a young child? Somebody's going to ask you, "What was this about observing girls in the shower?" Is there any possibility that he himself might have been abused in some way?

Comment

Before submitting this transcript for publication, we asked some experienced Board examiners to give us their impressions. Of eight examiners who did so, five gave the candidate an overall grade of Fail, and two gave a Condition (leaning toward Pass); only one gave this candidate an outright Pass. Of course, the two mock examiners agreed to pass the candidate by the narrowest of margins.

Although our sample size is small, we believe that it represents fairly the spectrum of opinion such an interview would generate on an actual Board examination. Numerous writers have observed how difficult it is to achieve consensus about an interview that is as marginal as this one. Most of our consultant examiners (though not all) thought that the candidate did better on the "patient-physician relationship" and "conduct of interview" sections. Several also noted the impression (from the written transcript, at any rate) that the mock examiners were unnecessarily cold and rigid.

This mock board was truly a harrowing experience, for the examiners as well as for the candidate. But it is a beautiful demonstration of what we have been trying to emphasize throughout *Boarding Time:* the value of the mock board exam. We subsequently learned that this candidate passed the actual Board examination on the first try!

Appendix A ——————————————

A Brief History of the ABPN

In 1910, the Flexner report changed forever the face of American medical education. But for a generation afterward the psychiatric profession still suffered an identity crisis. We no longer called ourselves *alienists,* but most medical schools offered little formal training in psychiatry. Few agreed as to what constituted adequate training in psychiatry. And until the 1930s any physician could be listed in the directory of the American Medical Association as a specialist in psychiatry—simply on request.

Most treatment modalities were nonspecific and unscientific. Competition for patients was intense and getting worse. Psychiatric patients were likely to seek their care from general physicians, faith healers, and Christian Science practitioners. Psychologists were still largely preoccupied with canine conditioning, so among specialists a psychiatrist of 50 years ago would feel a competitive threat most keenly from neurologists. Thus, with the formation of specialty societies in full swing by the late 1920s, one of the driving forces that eventually led to the formation of the ABPN was fear—the fear that if the psychiatrists did not do it, the neurologists would. If this happened, the argument ran, the neurologists would gain control of the patient population and, ultimately, of the mental health profession. Clearly, time was of the essence.

In the late 1920s, Adolph Meyer urged the formation of an organization to examine candidates, but it required several years of rumination by the American Medical Association, the American Psychiatric Association, and other medical organizations before the American Psychiatric Association approved the Board as a certifying body in 1933. In short order, it was also sanctioned by the American Medical Association and the American Neurological Association. (The American Academy of Neurology joined as the fourth cosponsor in 1974.)

The joint Board first met in 1934. Neurologists and psychiatrists were equally represented; this practice continues today, although the Board has been expanded to 16 members. Some discussion ensued regarding the choice of name. Because then, as now, psychiatrists could claim superior numbers nationally, they gained pride of place, as opposed to the alphabetical approach (favored by the neurologists). It was also decided to award separate certificates for psychiatry and neurology. This was a second victory for the psychiatrists, who now felt assured they would gain control of training and eventually, they hoped, of the vast pool of mental health patients.

The first examination was given in June of 1935. Thirty-one candidates sat for an exam that combined essays with oral examinations. Certificates were awarded to 22 examinees. It is not recorded whether those who failed subsequently reapplied.

The Contemporary ABPN

For many years, the ABPN has been under the jurisdiction of the American Board of Medical Specialties, the umbrella group that maintains standards for all medical specialty boards and approves the establishment of new boards. The intervening half century has witnessed a number of other changes, most of which work to the advantage of the candidate. Written exams, introduced in 1965, have been seriously used as a screening device since 1967. Now, first-time candidates can select the site they prefer for Part I, and they no longer must wait 2 years after completing residency to take it. (In fact, in response to requests from candidates and training directors, the Part I written examination was recently moved to the fall of each year, just a few months after most candidates finish their training.) After passing Part I, they now have 6 years to complete Part II successfully; now three failures, not two, on Part II mandate retaking Part I. Candidates are currently required to interview only one psychiatric patient; examining a live neurology patient and oral questioning by neurologists are but fading memories. Today, technology supplements human effort: a videotape has replaced one of the patient interviews, and computerization has affected all phases of the operation.

In the 50-plus years since the Board examination began, its mission has remained essentially the same. Here is the most recent statement of that mission, paraphrased from the ABPN publication *Information for Applicants:*

1. To describe the knowledge and skills required by physicians who would specialize in evaluating and treating psychiatric and/or neurological patients
2. To set standards for such knowledge and skills
3. To write and administer exams that will measure such knowledge and skills

4. To evaluate and improve the certification process
5. To help set standards for residency training
6. To issue certificates to successful candidates
7. To publish lists of those who have been certified
8. To inform the public about the activities of the Board
9. To participate in the American Board of Medical Specialties

Examination Content and Format

For 30 years after its birth, the Board examination remained essentially an oral affair. But by the mid-1960s the logistics of the oral exams had been complicated by several developments, including increasing numbers of candidates, an explosion of scientific information pertaining to psychiatry, and the persistent desire for testing procedures that are fair. It seemed clear that a written exam was needed.

During its more than 25 years of use, the all-written, more theoretical Part I has come to serve as a screening device for the more practical (and vastly more complicated and expensive to administer) Part II. Despite the oral exam's potential for emotional trauma, Part I is seen by many as the real barrier to certification. This effect may be partly psychological. As Greenblatt et al. (1977) noted, "A candidate who passes the written exam [on the first try] is much more likely to persist in the examination process and become a diplomate of the Board than one who initially fails Part I" (p. 1260). In that study, 88% of psychiatrists who passed Part I on the first try—but only 12% of those who initially failed Part I—went on to become Board certified within 4 years.

For candidates in psychiatry, Part I of the exam covers both neurology and psychiatry. The neurology section includes

- Clinical neurology
- Neuroanatomy
- Neuropathology
- Neuropharmacology
- Clinical diagnostic procedures, including questions on
    Cerebrospinal fluid
    Neuro-ophthalmology
    Electroencephalography
    Neuroimaging
- Therapy and management of patients with neurologic disorders

The psychiatric section covers

- Normal and abnormal growth and development through the life cycle
- Biological dimensions of psychiatry
- Psychosocial dimensions of psychiatry
- Clinical psychiatry
        Phenomenology
        Diagnosis
        Treatment

Table A–1. Candidates for psychiatry Boards, 1968–1994

Year	Took Part I	Passed	% Pass	Took Part II	Passed	% Pass
1968	966	777	80	313	186	59
1969	850	627	74	846	523	62
1970	887	562	63	943	624	66
1971	874	563	64	689	421	61
1972	779	500	64	874	537	61
1973	930	598	64	671	416	62
1974	1270	803	63	863	513	59
1975	1784	1164	65	1182	675	57
1976	1730	1473	85	1767	1086	61
1977	1469	1215	83	2027	1200	59
1978	1696	1394	82	1916	1110	58
1979	1672	1337	80	2145	1260	59
1980	1613	1299	81	2160	1227	57
1981	1228	1004	82	1883	1087	58
1982	1354	968	71	1728	932	54
1983	1359	953	70	1856	987	53
1984	1277	661	52	1559	857	55
1985	1588	843	53	1180	661	56
1986	1738	1036	60	1426	815	57
1987	1670	921	55	1403	779	56
1988	1787	1079	60	1434	881	60
1989	1946	1203	62	1560	930	60
1990	2108	1244	59	1629	967	59
1991	2422	1406	58	1881	1130	60
1992	2974	1788	60	2051	1256	61
1993	2982	1681	56	2671	1640	61
1994	2923	1829	63	2396	1467	61

Passing Part I is the only way a candidate can qualify to take Part II. This qualification is good for 6 years or three attempts to pass Part II, whichever occurs first. Any candidate who fails Part II on three occasions or who allows the 6 years to elapse without passing it must then retake the Part I examination. Table A–1 shows the numbers of candidates who have taken Part I and Part II over the past quarter century.

After passing Part I, you will be scheduled for a Part II examination that will take place within 1 year. Because of complicated logistics and limited space, you will not be able to select the date and site for your Part II examination. However, regionalized exams do keep your travel at a minimum.

In 1995, exams were given four times. In successive years, staff expect that three times a year will once again become the norm. Exams are given on each coast, as well as in the Midwest. The exam locations are moved around from year to year, so as not to place too great a burden on any one metropolitan area. One of these three exams is so large (roughly 1,100 candidates, of whom 75% are psychiatrists) that only five major cities can accommodate it. These centers are New York, Chicago, Philadelphia, Boston, and Washington, DC. The remaining exams, each of which comprises about 500 candidates (375 psychiatrists), are distributed around the country on a geographic basis. This gives examinees (and examiners) the chance to work close to home.

Appendix B ————————————————

Board Eligibility: U.S. and Canadian Trainees

The ABPN currently issues eight types of certificate: General Psychiatry, Child and Adolescent Psychiatry, Neurology, Neurology with Special Qualification in Child Neurology and Added Qualifications in Addiction Psychiatry, Clinical Neurophysiology, Forensic Psychiatry, and Geriatric Psychiatry. To hold more than one of these certificates, a candidate must be examined independently for each. Most of this book is concerned exclusively with the certificate in general psychiatry, the most frequently issued of these certificates.

Board Eligibility

To be allowed to take the examination in general psychiatry, you must meet these requirements:

1. You must have an unlimited license to practice medicine in a state, commonwealth, or territory of the United States or in a province of Canada. You must submit a copy of this license and of your current registration with your Part I application. After you have passed Part II, you will have to submit another copy of your license to practice medicine, including its date of expiration, before your certificate will be issued. This recent change is to assure the Board that your license has not elapsed since the time you first applied to take Part I.

2. You may apply for certification only after you have completed your training in an approved residency program. (You will find a listing of approved programs in the most recent issue of the *Directory of Graduate Medical Education Programs,* which is published by the American Medical Association.)
3. You must have successfully completed the training requirements specified by the ABPN. Either of two basic patterns may apply:

- *Four-year program.* If yours was a 4-year residency program, at least 4 months of the first year must have been devoted to the general medical care of adults or children. That means 4 months of internal medicine, pediatrics, or family medicine.
- *Three-year program.* If you graduated from an approved 3-year residency you must also have had a PGY-1 (first postgraduate year) of approved training that emphasizes general medical care. If you are a recent graduate, there are two principal ways you could have fulfilled your PGY-1 year of nonpsychiatric training: the categorical and the transitional programs. These have both been sanctioned by the Accreditation Council for Graduate Medical Education (ACGME) since July 1982.

Categorical programs are actually the first of a 4-year period of specialty training. During the first year, there is at least 4 months of work in one of the primary care specialties (pediatrics, internal medicine, or family practice).

Transitional programs are only a year long and involve a variety of medical specialty services. They are approximately equivalent to the mixed or rotating internships of years ago. A number of hospitals that do not have longer-term residency training programs offer transitional programs.

If you have specific questions about your training program, you should write to the Board to inquire (American Board of Psychiatry and Neurology, 500 Lake Cook Road, Suite 335, Deerfield, IL 60015). If you completed residency before 1976, special rules may apply, so it is important that you contact the Board with specific questions.

If you are a Doctor of Osteopathic Medicine (D.O.) and a graduate of a residency program approved by the ACGME, you can apply to take the exam if you have also completed an ACGME-approved PGY-1 year of training. The ABPN does not accept osteopathic internships as fulfilling the PGY-1 requirement and will not accept an osteopathic residency in psychiatry.

Because the details of the requirements for all applicants may change from one year to the next, be sure that you use the most recent ABPN information when you evaluate your own eligibility. If you are unsure, write for help.

Beginning with those entering their residency training as of July 1, 1997, all physicians must have completed 4 years of ACGME-approved postgraduate training, including a PGY-1 year as described above, to be eligible to take the general adult psychiatry Board exams. This holds true for all international graduates and includes those trained in Canada. Whether a Canadian license will continued to be accepted by the ABPN was not resolved at the time of this writing.

Appendix C —————————————————

Board Eligibility: International Trainees

U ntil the end of the twentieth century, special rules for eligibility apply if you received your psychiatric training outside the United States or Canada. Furthermore, the rules that apply to you depend on where and when you trained. One requirement that applies to everyone is that you must have a nonrestricted license to practice medicine in a state, commonwealth, or territory of the United States or in a province of Canada. Another is that all international trainees (including those who trained in the United Kingdom) must complete a year of primary care training in the United States or Canada. This means that you must fulfill the same PGY-1 (first postgraduate year) requirements that apply to graduates of U.S. and Canadian programs. The only exception is for those whose psychiatric training was taken in its entirety in one country (United Kingdom or any country outside the United States). Then, if you also have a national certificate in psychiatry (see below) from the country in which you trained, the requirement for a year of primary care training may be waived.

Note that, beginning with those entering their residency training as of July 1, 1997, all physicians must have completed 4 years of postgraduate training approved by the Accreditation Council for Graduate Medical Education (ACGME), including a PGY-1 year as described previously, to be eligible to take the general adult psychiatry Board exams. (Similar rules will apply for other certificates issued by the ABPN.) This holds true for all international graduates, including those trained in the United Kingdom, Israel, South Africa, and Australia–New Zealand. Credit will not be given for training in programs that the

ACGME does not accredit. Among other effects, in any future edition of this book this appendix will become unnecessary.

United Kingdom

If you trained in the United Kingdom and you began your residency training on or after July 1, 1976, you can receive 1 year of credit for each year of training in an approved program. To receive credit for 2 or 3 years, at least 2 of them must have been in the same program. An approved training program is one that has been sanctioned by the Visiting Inspecting Specialty Committee in Psychiatry of the Royal College of Physicians.

The details of the training program and the dates during which it was undertaken must be forwarded to the ABPN; this task is the responsibility of the applicant. Your program's training director must certify in a letter that you were involved in the program full time during the dates specified.

If you completed your psychiatric residency in the United Kingdom before July 1, 1976, you must follow the rules for non–United Kingdom trainees given below. If your training does not fall exactly into any of these categories, you should write to the ABPN. The Credentials Committee, which will rule on your application on an individual basis, will be better able to decide if you enclose as much documentation and detail about your training as possible. Regardless of when you trained, you must also have completed an approved year of primary care training in the United States or Canada.

Non–United Kingdom International Trainees

If you trained outside the United Kingdom, you must have had full-time specialty training that is equivalent to U.S. standards in terms of time and content. You must also be certified in psychiatry by the country in which you took your psychiatric training. This certificate must have been issued within 7 years of the date of your application. If the certificate was issued earlier, it must be supplemented by a year of clinical psychiatric practice in a setting where your professional work was observed by two physicians who hold psychiatry certificates from the ABPN. These two psychiatrists must submit letters of sponsorship to the Board on your behalf.

At present, only four countries have national certificates in psychiatry that are unequivocally recognized and accepted by the ABPN. Those countries (and the names of their respective certificates) are

- Australia and New Zealand (Member of The Royal Australia and New Zealand College of Psychiatry)
- Israel (Specialty Certification of The Scientific Counsel of The Israel Medical Association)
- South Africa (Fellowship of The Faculty of Psychiatry of The College of Medicine of South Africa)
- United Kingdom (Member of The Royal College of Psychiatry)

The Credentials Committee of the ABPN may also accept certificates from other countries. However, the process of acceptance is not automatic, and an application must be made in writing to the Board.

Until around the year 2000, the real issue for international trainees is the PGY-1 year of training. In essence, no such training taken outside the United States or Canada will be accepted by the Board. Exceptions may be granted by the Credentials Committee for applicants with truly outstanding and equivalent training, but this is unusual.

Appendix D ——————————

Measuring Success

How well does the exam test what clinical psychiatrists need to know? Through the years, this controversial question has generated far more heat than light. Neither of the two qualities that must be addressed by those who construct examinations has been adequately explored for the psychiatry Boards. Those qualities are validity and reliability.

There are essentially no data that can help us determine validity, which we will define here as the exam's ability to measure a psychiatrist's clinical adequacy. This lack is largely because we don't know how to define *adequacy* in any but the broadest and most subjective of terms. Therefore, we have no way of correlating success on Part II of the ABPN with clinical performance. However, the reason that the ABPN clings so tenaciously to this examination format (it is the only specialty board that continues to use actual patients) is the general opinion that this process, expensive and time-consuming as it is, provides the best guarantee that certificate holders will be competent to evaluate and manage patients. Several years ago this assessment was vetted by American Psychiatric Association members, who overwhelmingly voted to retain the oral, live patient format.

How reliable is the examination process? By reliability, we mean consistency in a test-retest situation. Again, few data are available. However, candidates who initially fail Part II are much more likely to fail it on a subsequent try. As of 1977, when the most recent data were published, only about half of all psychiatry candidates passed both parts of the Boards on their first try. Greenblatt et al. (1977) commented on this statistic: "This may mean that the exams are deficient, that candidates are insufficiently prepared, or that the exams, despite an admitted need for further improvement, do serve to maintain essential professional standards by not permitting overly easy access to specialty status" (p. 1260).

McDermott et al. (1991) evaluated the reliability of the Part II examination process by studying interexaminer consistency for 1,422 candidates. Overall, in 67% of examinations there was perfect agreement as to the candidate's performance. That is, the two examiners initially each gave the candidate the same Pass, Condition, or Fail grade on either the patient interview or videotape examination. There were minor disagreements (Pass-Condition or Fail-Condition) for 26% of candidates, and major disagreement (Fail-Pass) for only 7% of candidates. The overall weighted kappa statistic was 0.56, which they judged to show fair to good agreement beyond chance. In a second report, these authors (McDermott et al. 1993) found that the examination process was stable across seasons of the year and different examination sites in the United States. They concluded: "There is no evidence that factors such as examiner fatigue to increasing experience influence interexaminer consistency" (p. 1079).

However, the authors did note with some concern that, the kappa statistic notwithstanding, the overall agreement was still only in the moderate range. In cases where the examiners disagreed, the disagreement was relatively minor nearly 80% of the time: a Condition combined with a Pass or Fail. Discussion (sometimes involving the senior examiner) usually resolved these disagreements with relative ease. But in the 7% where there was a major disagreement between examiners, a thorough review (with participation of the senior examiner) of the candidate's entire performance was usually necessary to make the final decision as to whether the deficiency was major or minor. Most of these major disagreements turned on the concern of one examiner about a specific act (omission or commission) on the part of the candidate.

Evaluating the Examination

Most examinees—80% or more (Naftulin et al. 1977)—say that the videotape exam is a useful learning and testing device. Because this testing modality has become a mainstay of the Part II examination, the ABPN clearly agrees with that assessment. Several factors contribute to its popularity:

1. It increases the efficiency of the exam because only one patient interview is required rather than two, thus halving the number of patients needed.
2. Candidates at any given half-day session see the same interview tape. Having stimulus data in common sets the stage for a more uniform, hence more reliable, examination.
3. It is easier for candidates and examiners alike to discuss a videotape, with the data already provided, than a live patient, with data collection depending on the vagaries of the clinical interview. However, this advantage is diminished by the fact that the videotape exam, which provides no oppor-

tunity to evaluate interaction with patients, is probably a less valid measure of clinical competence.

Are the exams deficient? Or, because all exams have their deficiencies, perhaps we should instead ask, How deficient are the exams? We do have some data concerning the concordance rate between the live patient and videotape sessions. These data were reported by Talbott (1983), who studied Pass-Condition-Fail rates for videotape and live patient exams in 2,236 candidates during the early 1980s. He defined concordance as either identical scores on both tests or as a Failure coupled with a Condition, which in practice results in failing Part II of the Boards. He defined nonconcordance as a Pass coupled with either a Failure or a Condition. (Because in practice a candidate who passes one portion of the exam and receives a Condition on the other will usually pass overall and be awarded a certificate, this definition produced a conservative estimate of concordance.)

Of all 2,236 candidates, 52% had identical grades, and 61% had concordant grades by the operational definition (Talbott 1983). Considering the fact that the two exam formats test somewhat different skills and carry different weights in the judgment of many examiners, Talbott stated that this concordance rate was acceptable. Of the 869 candidates who had nonconcordant grades, 303 (35%) had grades that were highly discordant (that is, they received a Pass on one exam and a Failure on the other). A candidate with dissimilar scores was twice as likely to have a higher score on the videotape session than on the patient interview.

The fact that the passing rate is higher on the videotape exam than on the patient interview (see Table D–1) suggests that examiners may tend to grade the videotape more liberally. Another possible explanation is that residency programs may better prepare their graduates to do well in the cognitive aspects of psychiatry than in the performance skills of patient interviewing. Still another has already been noted: it is easier to discuss a case for which the data are already

Table D–1. Comparison of videotape and live patient exams

	Live patient			
Videotape	Pass	Condition	Fail	Total
Pass	921	348	224	1493
Condition	218	149	127	494
Fail	79	75	95	249
Total	1218	572	446	2236

Source. Data from Talbott (1983).

provided. In any event, because a Pass on one section of the exam coupled with a Condition on the other usually results in passing overall, the use of the video-tape exam may work to the advantage of some candidates.

In summing up the distinctions between these two exam formats, Talbott (1983) noted that the patient interview should let the examiner learn whether "the candidate can set the patient at ease, establish good therapeutic contact, maintain interpersonal relatedness, elicit pertinent information, monitor coun-tertransferential reactions, ask direct and open-ended as well as sympathetic and productive questions, and shift modes as warranted in the interview" (p. 892). On the other hand, the videotape interview "can obviously ascertain none of these, but instead should concentrate directly on the cognitive aspects of the clinical problems presented (e.g., the mental status, diagnosis, and therapy)" (p. 892). McDermott et al. (1993) remarked that "the total kappa statistics for the live patient and videotape formats were identical (kappa = 0.56)."

As you can see from this brief review, there are still many unanswered ques-tions concerning the validity and reliability of the entire psychiatry examination. Apart from the two studies cited, these questions remain largely unexamined for Part II. The ABPN is working on several other research projects designed to ex-amine, among other matters, the efficiency of different grading systems.

Passing the exam depends almost wholly on the subjective judgment of the examiners, who, although they are guided by the carefully thought out principles that underlie the exam, must in the end base their decisions principally on accu-mulated years of clinical experience. Although this process may be seen as a weakness, it is also one of the towering strengths of the examination process. We believe that this examination is a good test of clinical competence; overall, it is a fair test. It is not a perfect test, but it is getting better. And it is the only test we have.

Appendix E

Suggestions for Further Reading

We have selected the books for this brief appendix not as required reading, but as supplements to DSM-IV and the texts we discussed in Chapter 2. We mention them because we believe that some candidates will want to delve deeper into certain topics, for more detailed information or for interest.

The Clinical Interview Using DSM-IV, by Ekkehard Othmer and Sieglinde C. Othmer, Washington, DC, American Psychiatric Press, 1994. Usefully keyed to DSM-IV, this text also offers a detailed program for learning clinical interview skills.

Clinical Psychiatry and the Law, by Robert I. Simon, Washington, DC, American Psychiatric Press, 1987. Each chapter discusses a different legal problem, any of which a psychiatrist might encounter during the course of a general clinical practice.

Diagnostic Interviewing, by Michel Hersen and Samuel M. Turner, New York, Plenum, 1985. This is a useful manual for clinicians who want to hone their interviewing skills.

DSM-IV Made Easy, by James Morrison, New York, Guilford, 1994. This new book offers simplified diagnostic criteria, case vignettes for over 100 mental disorders, and discussions of all adult DSM-IV disorders.

The First Interview, by James Morrison, New York, Guilford, 1995. This book covers principles derived from results of scientific studies of interview technique. It was recently updated and keyed to DSM-IV.

Manual of Clinical Psychopharmacology, 2nd Edition, by Alan F. Schatzberg and Jonathan O. Cole, Washington, DC, American Psychiatric Press, 1991. Most candidates seem to be well grounded in psychopharmacology. However, you will probably want something to serve as a touchstone for this important area. This volume will serve admirably.

Medical Letter. Published biweekly, this is an excellent resource for newly released medications. Available by subscription or in medical libraries.

The Practitioner's Guide to Psychoactive Drugs, 3rd Edition, by Alan J. Gelenberg, Ellen L. Bassuck, and Stephen C. Schoonover, New York, Plenum, 1991. An excellent concise reference.

Treatment of Psychiatric Disorders, 2nd Edition, edited by Glen O. Gabbard, Washington, DC, American Psychiatric Press, 1995. This two-volume book covers a great deal of ground and makes an effort to remain uncommitted to any one therapeutic point of view.

Because of the variety of therapeutic systems and the difficulty of learning psychotherapy by the book, we hardly dare recommend a textbook on psychotherapy. Most comprehensive textbooks of psychiatry provide many opportunities to study different therapeutic systems. Candidates may nonetheless want to consult books on the brief psychotherapies, interpersonal psychotherapies, cognitive therapy, family therapy, and behavior modification therapy, as well as traditional psychodynamic psychotherapy.

Surveys of candidates consistently show that journal article reading is the least useful thing they have done to prepare for Board examinations. However, you will probably feel more comfortable if you keep up with several psychiatric periodicals. We favor (in alphabetical order): *The American Journal of Psychiatry, Archives of General Psychiatry, The British Journal of Psychiatry, Comprehensive Psychiatry,* and *The Journal of Nervous and Mental Disease.* Any subject that becomes important in psychiatry sooner or later makes its way into these main journals.

Appendix F ————————————————

Robins-Guze Criteria for Psychiatric Diagnosis

1. *Clinical description.* This is the essential first step in formulating any valid diagnosis. It is classical, descriptive medicine that is based on the clinical observation of many patients. The clinical picture may be dominated by a single principal feature or by a collection of characteristics that are associated with one another in a syndrome. The clinical description includes symptoms, signs, history, and demographic data.

2. *Follow-up study.*[1] Apart from the initial clinical description, and in lieu of known etiologies and diagnostic laboratory testing procedures, this phase has been the key to the formulation of valid psychiatric diagnoses. Although two patients with the same illness don't always have the same outcome, markedly different outcomes suggest that they may have different illnesses. At follow-up of patients in any diagnostic group, a high incidence of change of diagnosis or a markedly heterogeneous outcome is cause for concern. Either finding suggests that the selection criteria or selection process must be further refined. The need for physicians to make predictions about the disorders they treat underscores the importance of the follow-up study in medicine.

3. *Delimitation from other disorders.* This is accomplished by developing exclusion criteria to ensure that the group studied is as homogeneous as possible.

————————————————

1 Robins and Guze (1970) originally listed step 2, follow-up study, in the fourth position. Because of its critical importance to psychiatry, we have relocated it. For similar reasons, we have placed laboratory studies last.

4. *Family study.* Whether because of heredity or environment, many psychiatric disorders run in families. So, if relatives of patients with disorder K also have disorder K, we consider it evidence that the diagnosis is valid.

5. *Laboratory studies.* These include chemical, radiologic, physiologic, and psychological tests in the living patient, as well as the results of autopsy examinations. As of this writing, laboratory tests still play a significant role in the description of few psychiatric disorders.

Appendix G

What About Recertification?

In the United States, the impetus toward recertification dates back well over half a century. The Commission on Medical Education of the American Association of Medical Colleges suggested in 1933 that "every physician may be required in the public interest to take continuation courses to ensure that his practice will be kept abreast of current methods of diagnosis and treatment" (Shore and Scheiber 1994, p. 255). In 1940, the commission followed up with the statement that "as the certifying boards become better established, and as they complete the examination of a large group of physicians already practicing the specialties, they may find it desirable to issue certificates that are valid for a stated period only" (Shore and Scheiber 1994, p. 255).

Then in 1973, the American Board of Medical Specialties passed a formal resolution on recertification:

> That ABMS adopt, in principle, and urge concurrence of its member boards with the policy that voluntary, periodic recertification of medical specialties become an integral part of all national medical specialty certification programs and, further, that ABMS establish a reasonable deadline when voluntary, periodic recertification of medical specialists will have become a standard policy of all member boards. (Shore and Scheiber 1994, p. 255)

After a national referendum, the American Psychiatric Association, in 1978, published its *Guidelines for Recertification,* which included the following eight items (Shore and Scheiber 1994, p. 13):

1. It must be a voluntary process.
2. There must be a set of options.

3. It expressed opposition to mandatory, externally evaluated examinations.
4. It should be open to uncertified psychiatrists.
5. Although there should be some amount of core material, allowance should be made for demonstrated competence in a psychiatrist's specific work area.
6. The process of certification should be a continuing one.
7. A variety of methods should be used, including continuing medical education, the American Psychiatric Association self-assessment program, and demonstration of competence through clinical work.
8. The document expressed opposition to double jeopardy for subspecialists.

In 1989, in a meeting of the ABPN to discuss certification and recertification, the Board took four far-reaching actions:

- It approved a 10-year, time-limited certificate for candidates certified after October 1994.
- It decided to consider moving the written examination closer to the completion of residency.
- It created an interorganizational task force on the psychiatry written examination.
- It initiated a formal evaluation process by creating an office of research and the position of research director.

As the result of these actions, the group stated that "the first recertification examination will be given no later than January 1, 2000" (Shore and Scheiber 1994, p. 11).

The Specter of Recertification

Now 1994 has come and gone, and lifetime certification has been replaced by recertification (called continuing certification by some) and lifetime learning. What promise do these innovations, which will become reality within just a few years, hold for our specialty?

A variety of options are spelled out by several authors in a 1994 book edited by Drs. James Shore and Stephen Scheiber: *Certification, Recertification, and Lifetime Learning in Psychiatry.* Here are a few of them:

- *Standard written examinations.* Like any currently used exam, these would have to be kept secret, making feedback to candidates difficult.
- *The essay.* Some authors believe that the written essay better allows practitioners to describe how psychotherapeutic and psychodynamic

concepts might be applied to a patient. There are, of course, serious problems of consistency in grading.

- *Take-home examinations that run on the physicians' microcomputers.* The American Board of Pediatrics has already experimented with this method.
- *Chart reviews of the candidate's own written records.* Used by the American Board of Family Practice as a screening test to take the recertification exam, the candidate selects charts from several categories and records data about many items. Failure to complete the computer database can result in ineligibility to take the recertification exam.
- *Patient and staff satisfaction.* Patients' and co-workers' attitudes toward a practitioner are obviously of relevance and interest to quality of clinical care. Methodology and validity could leave much to be desired, however.
- *Videotaped office visits.* Evaluation by this method, which involves the scoring of one of the candidate's office visits against protocols, has been pioneered in Australia.
- *The "standardized patient."* This method, which achieves standardization by using simulated patients, has been used by the Medical Council of Canada. It can be made reliable with adequate training of the "patient"; it cannot, apparently, be made inexpensive.

The Crystal Ball

The foregoing are only some of the options. What form is recertification likely to assume in the coming century? In 1994, six leaders in American psychiatry began meeting to discuss this question. The panel, which comprised three directors of the ABPN, two appointees of the American Psychiatric Association, and an appointee of the American Academy of Child and Adolescent Psychiatry, was chaired by Kenneth Altshuler, M. D. When its task is completed, this committee will report its recommendations to the full Board of the ABPN.

As of this writing, the answers are not yet clear; indeed, they may not be clear for some time. Here, however, based on a question-and-answer feature by Stephen Scheiber, M.D., in the American Association of Directors of Psychiatric Residency Training Newsletter (1994), are our best impressions of the directions recertification will (or won't) take:

Continuing certification, which will become known as Part III of the Boards, will be a reality by the year 2000. Diplomates whose certificates are issued after September 1994 (these will all be 10-year, time-limited certificates) will be required to take the new exam. But others who desire recertification will probably be allowed to do so, also.

Although the exact form this exam will take is not clear as of this writing, some variation of one of the options mentioned above will almost surely be used. There are plans to link it, in some as-yet unspecified manner, to continuing education. It may be developed along modular lines, with clinicians being allowed to select from a list of topics or areas of their special expertise. These modules will emphasize recent advances in clinical psychiatry. They could be based in part on the practice guidelines that the American Psychiatric Association has recently begun to publish sporadically in the *American Journal of Psychiatry.*

This exam will not focus on the basic sciences of psychiatry, and there will be no minor component in neurology. As of this writing, there is only a remote chance that Part III will be given as an oral exam. This is due to the expense and the vast administrative network that such an exam would entail, not to mention the fact that Board-certified psychiatrists have already experienced that ordeal.

As with Part II, the candidate would have to submit documentation of an unlimited license to practice medicine to be eligible to take this exam. Unlike Part II, the pass rate is expected to be high—90% or greater. As Dr. Scheiber explained in a telephone interview (August 1994), "The intent is not to exclude, but to ascertain whether the psychiatrist has been keeping up with advances in the clinical practice of psychiatry."

References

Scheiber SC: Q&A: Recertification. American Association of directors of Psychiatric Residency Training Newsletter 22(summer):11, 15, 1994

American Psychiatric Association: Diagnostic and Statistical Manual of Mental Disorders, 3rd Edition. Washington, DC, American Psychiatric Association, 1980

American Psychiatric Association: Diagnostic and Statistical Manual of Mental Disorders, 3rd Edition, Revised. Washington, DC, American Psychiatric Association, 1987

American Psychiatric Association: Diagnostic and Statistical Manual of Mental Disorders, 4th Edition. Washington, DC, American Psychiatric Association, 1994

Andreasen NC: Thought, language, and communication disorders, I: clinical assessment, definition of terms, and evaluation of their reliability. Arch Gen Psychiatry 36:1315–1321, 1979a

Andreasen NC: Thought, language, and communication disorders, II: diagnostic significance. Arch Gen Psychiatry 36:1325–1330, 1979b

Brown BM: An examinee's perspective on board certification. Am J Psychiatry 134:1261–1264, 1977

Eddy DM, Clanton CH: The art of diagnosis. N Engl J Med 306:1263–1268, 1982

Eveloff HH, McCreary CP: The attitudes of patients and their trainee therapists toward participation in psychiatric board examinations. Am J Psychiatry 129:616–620, 1972

Galen RS, Gambino SR: Beyond Normality: The Predictive Value and Efficiency of Medical Diagnoses. New York, Wiley, 1975

Gauron EF, Dickinson JK: Diagnostic decision making in psychiatry, II: diagnostic styles. Arch Gen Psychiatry 14:233–237, 1966

Greenblatt M, Carew J, Pierce CM: Success rates in psychiatry and neurology certification examinations. Am J Psychiatry 134:1259–1261, 1977

Haas AP, Hendin H, Singer P: Psychodynamic and structured interviewing: issues of validity. Compr Psychiatry 28:40–53, 1987

Kaplan HI, Sadock BJ, Grebb JA: Kaplan and Sadock's Synopsis of Psychiatry, 7th Edition. Baltimore, MD, Williams & Wilkins, 1994

Lipp MR: Experiences of psychiatry board exam casualties: a survey report. Am J Psychiatry 133:279–283, 1976

Maleson FG, Fink PJ, Field HL: Board certification anxiety. Am J Psychiatry 137:837–840, 1980

Maxmen JS: Essential Psychopathology. New York, WW Norton, 1986

McDermott JF Jr, Tanguay PE, Scheiber SC, et al: Reliability of the part II board certification examination in psychiatry: interexaminer consistency. Am J Psychiatry 148:1672–1674, 1991

McDermott JF Jr, Tanguay PE, Scheiber SC, et al: Reliability of the part II board certification examination in psychiatry: examination stability. Am J Psychiatry 150:1077–1080, 1993

Morrison JR, Muñoz RA: 650 private psychiatric patients. J Clin Psychiatry 40:114–116, 1979

Naftulin DH, Wolkon GH, Donnelly FA, et al: A comparison of videotaped and live patient interview examinations and written examinations in psychiatry. Am J Psychiatry 134:1093–1097, 1977

Napoliello MJ: From board candidate to rookie examiner. Am J Psychiatry 134:1264–1266, 1977

Othmer E, DeSouza C: A screening test for somatization disorder (hysteria). Am J Psychiatry 142:1146–1149, 1985

Quick SK, Robinowitz CB: Examination success and opinions of American Board of Psychiatry and Neurology certification. Am J Psychiatry 138:340–344, 1981

Robins E, Guze SB: Establishment of diagnostic validity in psychiatric illness: its application to schizophrenia. Am J Psychiatry 126:983–987, 1970

Robins LN, Helzer JE, Weissman MM, et al: Lifetime prevalence of specific psychiatric disorders in three sites. Arch Gen Psychiatry 41:949–958, 1984

Rosen H, Cohen LB, Schwartz L, et al: Response of patients to participation in psychiatry board examinations. Am J Psychiatry 136:330–332, 1979

Rosenhan DL: On being sane in insane places. Science 179:250–258, 1973

Rudy LH, Kulieke MJ: Reasons given for success after initial failure on the American Board of Psychiatry and Neurology Part II examination. Am J Psychiatry 138:1612–1615, 1981

Shore JH, Scheiber SC (eds): Certification, Recertification and Lifetime Learning in Psychiatry. Washington, DC, American Psychiatric Association, 1994

Talbott JA: Is the "live patient" interview on the boards necessary? Am J Psychiatry 140:890–893, 1983

Hales RE, Yudofsky SC, Talbott JA (eds): The American Psychiatric Press Textbook of Psychiatry, 2nd Edition. Washington, DC, American Psychiatric Press, 1994

Index

215